HEAL YOUR WOUND

A Doctor's Guide for Hard-to-Heal Wounds

ALVIN MAY, MD

HEAL YOUR WOUND

A Doctor's Guide for Hard-to-Heal Wounds

Alvin May MD

ISBN: 978-1-962976-00-8

Illustrated by Aveliya Design
Editorial Design: Luca Funari

Printed by Jackson Clara Publishing in the USA
www.JacksonClaraPublishing.com

Scan or visit:

www.WoundWise.com

for more valuable
wound healing resources

DEDICATION

This book is dedicated to my family:

To a wife who combines a good heart, a warm smile, and belief in self to do absolutely amazing things. You are a constant reminder that compassion and consistency both open hearts and move mountains.

My three beautiful daughters whose very presence reminds me that you put magic into the world when you continue to learn, grow, and evolve as a person, no matter your age.

Amazing parents whose love, guidance, and support helped lay a wonderful life path for me to follow.

And grandparents and forebearers whose words of wisdom, sacrifices, lives, and legacies continue to be an inspiration for me to this day.

You all mean the world to me. I cannot thank you enough for your unwavering love and support.

I would be remiss if I did not also thank the many teachers, colleagues, and mentors who helped cultivate the information and perspective needed to write this book. Finally, to the hundreds of nurses and caregivers with whom I have worked who do the real "heavy lifting" in the world of wound care. Your work is invaluable.

FOREWORD

Every wound tells a story. The stories of chronic wounds are ones of long roads with twists and turns, setbacks, and sometimes even dead ends. The responsibility of wound care professionals like me is to help navigate these challenges, hopefully finding closure for these difficult-to-heal wounds and relief for the patients who have them.

Though not a wound patient myself just yet, my personal journey with long-term wound care is also a long one. It began just after I completed medical school during my years in training to become a general surgeon. It was during this surgical training that I developed the skills necessary to perform various operations, along with fostering the skills to manage and treat the wounds that result from those surgical procedures. It was there that I began to learn from a pair of wound and ostomy nurses about how to approach, foster, and care for chronic wounds as well as the patients who have them. While learning the craft of being a physician and surgeon, I also received a masterclass in the art of wound care. Little did I know then that long-term wound care would become a passion of mine—and, eventually, my career—influencing my life in so many unexpected ways.

In my early years of practice as a general surgeon, my grandmother (who at the age of 100 years had almost convinced us she might live forever) finally began to show the generally expected signs of her age right before our eyes. Grandma has since passed on, but she was a remarkable woman who radiated grace, energy, and vivacity. As a lifelong teacher, she had always emphasized education and was much of the reason why I pursued academics so diligently and ultimately chose a career in medicine. It was around her 102nd birthday, and it seemed like overnight that we noticed the change. Suddenly, she started facing many more of the common challenges that come with aging. It was amazing, though, because even as her health eventually declined, her mental acuity remained intact. While my grandmother's mental fortitude gave us more time with her, it was difficult seeing her come to the painful realization that her body was failing her. She struggled with generalized weakness, weight loss, limited mobility, and leg swelling as well as a list of other medical issues that made her activities of daily living much more challenging.

One day, while moving from her bed to a chair, my grandmother suffered a skin tear on her lower leg—a condition in which the top layer of skin, known as the epithelium, is torn away from the underlying skin, resulting in an open wound. Typically, skin tears can heal within a few days in a young, healthy person. However, in my grandmother's case, the wound persisted for weeks and months due to the swelling in her legs caused by underlying heart failure. While home for the holidays that year, I remember sitting down next to my grandmother. I always loved spending time with her.

She was lying in her bed watching television, and I recall her looking up at me and asking, "Baby, why won't this heal?" as she pointed at her lower leg.

I looked down at the swollen leg and the drainage-stained bandage covering the wound below it. The skin over her shins was shiny and stretched thin from all the excess fluid in her legs. I knew that the swollen state of her legs was compressing and narrowing the vessels within the leg that should have been bringing vital blood flow to the wound. I knew that the excess fluid in the legs was under pressure and looking for a way out, causing excessive drainage. I knew that the excessive fluid draining onto the skin around the wound would damage the skin and prevent the wound from filling in.

I took her hand in mine and replied, "This kind of thing gets harder as we get older, but we can heal this."

And heal it we did. By diligently elevating her legs while she was in bed or in a chair (the places where she spent the majority of her time at that point), we were able to use gravity to drain the excess fluid from her legs. We employed a special positioner to lift her leg in such a way as to draw excess fluid away from the wound to decrease damaging wound drainage and improve blood flow to the wound itself.

As I look back, it's amazing to think how far medical advancement had come over the 100-plus years of my grandmother's lifespan. Surely, many of those advancements even helped her to live longer than folks having the same medical issues only 20 or 30 years prior. Congestive heart failure and an irregular heartbeat were regular issues, to be sure. The care she received from her personal doctor of many years, Dr. Cohen, was her key to accessing the medical advancements that granted her more years and more cherished moments with her family and loved ones. On the flipside, Grandma faced the challenge of living with all the complications that came with this extended lease on life, including wound care issues.

It was through this experience that I became familiar with the anxiety, confusion, and frustration that surround wounds that inexplicably will not heal. It's a feeling well-known to so many chronic wound patients, their caregivers, and—if you're reading this book—I'm guessing you as well. It was during this period that I began dedicating more and more of my time and medical practice to the treatment and healing of chronic wounds. Today, it is by far the majority of what I do day-to-day. In my practice, I have encountered countless wound patients. While I care for and counsel patients and their caregivers daily, I'm frequently struck by how often someone has had their wound for weeks, months, or even years but doesn't understand why their wound persists or what things they can do to accelerate their wound healing.

While my patients receive care from a specialized wound doctor highly trained in their field, I realize that not all patients have access to such a specialist. That lack of universal access to care is why I created this book—to provide you with an easily accessible, easily digestible handbook that combines information, experience, and insights about wound care into a simple, easy-to-use guide.

I hear about the frustrations that come with delayed wound healing on a daily basis. My experience over the years tells me that patients often simply do not understand the fundamentals of chronic wound healing. I cannot tell you how often I hear from a patient or their family member during an initial consultation, "Is that what's going on? We've been dealing with this wound for I don't know how long. No one ever explained it to us like that."

Patients often just assume that their wound will heal like every other scratch and cut they had before in their life. Unfortunately, with chronic wounds, assumptions like this only add to frustration and delayed healing. Probably even more insidious, though, is that patients overlook or simply ignore the critical role that small, non-medical actions can play in wound healing.

Healing for a chronic wound can be slow and confusing and stressful, which is exactly why it often requires specialized insight and support of a wound care professional. Without this specialized insight and support, like a small child who doesn't know any better, we find ourselves helpless. I get it—it's human nature to ignore what we don't understand. Under all the medical jargon, unpronounceable medications, and never-ending tests, it can be difficult to keep up with what your doctor is saying, much less understand why the stubborn wound on your leg simply will not heal. Similarly, it may be overwhelming to try to understand why the high blood sugars of your diabetes have anything to do with that unsightly wound on your foot. And what happens when we don't understand? We disengage, we wait to see what will happen, and we don't act. Don't worry though, it's not just you; it's human nature. But I want to help you change all that. Together, let's find the steps you need to take to heal your wound.

Okay, so we see the problem. Now, let's fix it. In this handbook, I will provide you with the fundamentals of chronic wounds and strategies that you can use in your everyday life to help heal them. Let's add this to what your doctor is doing and unlock the other half of healing: the power of patient-driven healing. I want to help you better understand your wound and the strategies that will help you heal your wound faster. I will present these chronic wound types in a systematic manner as well as the conditions that give rise to them in a language and through concepts that you can relate to.

For instance, we can all understand the experience of stepping on a LEGO brick barefoot. Ouch! The tiny LEGO brick causes intense pain because your body's weight is now focused on a very small area (where the LEGO is embedded) rather than being spread out over the entire area of your foot. This is exactly what happens with pressure ulcers (or "bedsores" as they were formerly called). If you are sitting or lying down for an extended period, small bony prominences like your heel bone or tailbone (we call these pressure points) act just like that LEGO—focusing a significant proportion of your body weight on a relatively small, specific area. So, if you are unable to move freely due to age, injury, or disability, this pressure can lead to pain and eventually to tissue damage and ulceration.

Let's try another example. Consider the experience of being stuck in traffic. We have all been there, right? And just as cars carry people along streets and highways to different destinations, blood carries oxygen through the vessels of the circulatory system to the various organs and tissues that need it. If there happens to be traffic on the way to your destination, then you won't arrive on time. Similarly, when blood is slow to reach its destination in the body—say, due to arterial narrowing or diabetes—life-giving oxygen doesn't make it to ulcers in time, which prevents them from healing.

By using relatable analogies like the ones above, you can gain a better understanding of how to approach, think about, and heal your chronic wounds.

These are the kinds of concepts I want to introduce you to in this book. First, we'll establish a foundation for understanding what causes these wounds. Once we understand *why* these wounds occur, then we will look at the strategies to overcome the barriers that are preventing you from healing your wound.

I wrote this book for you to use in one of two ways: either as a textual overview to walk you through the world of wound healing or as a reference manual so that you can look up and better understand specific topics in wound care. After reading this book, you will be able to look at your wound, understand the factors that led to it, and know what actions you can take to help reverse the damages of your wound. Join me on this journey toward patient-driven healing.

DISCLAIMER

This handbook was written to be a resource to empower patients and caregivers navigating the challenging journey of chronic wound management—to foster hope, healing, and a sense of control. However, this handbook is in no way a substitute for professional medical advice. It is not a medical textbook or a medical reference. Similarly, the publisher does not provide medical advice or guidance. The information in this book is intended to be used and *must* be used for informational purposes only. You should always consult your personal healthcare professional for guidance on the specific management of your wound care needs and healthcare issues. Please independently verify any information contained within this book and consult with your medical provider prior to implementing any interventions mentioned herein into the care plan that you implement for yourself or provide for someone else.

This information is provided and intended to be used as general-purpose, topic-based enrichment. The content of this book should only be used as an adjunct to and in conjunction with the instructions, advice, and recommendations of your healthcare provider based on your personal medical history and your specific clinical needs and circumstances. All patient names mentioned in this handbook have been changed to protect their privacy.

TABLE OF CONTENTS

The Road Ahead on the Wound Healing Journey

If you're reading this book, you already understand what I am about to say. Chronic wounds can be complex, sometimes even downright head-scratching. There is simply no denying it. But the complexity of these wounds does not mean there's no hope for healing them. Yes, these kinds of wounds may be a challenge, but treating them does not have to be overwhelming. Chronic wounds are most often related to a medical condition like diabetes or circulation problems or may possibly be related to a physical issue like limited mobility from a recent surgery, a stroke, or simply the weakness that comes with age.

I will walk you through the concepts that lead to chronic wounds and make them difficult to heal. In my career, I have treated thousands of these wounds and explained these same concepts just as many times to patients like you. I will bring all of that experience to bear to help you understand and appreciate the intricate nature of healing your chronic wound. From pressure ulcers to diabetic foot ulcers and venous leg ulcers to non-healing surgical wounds, each wound has its own unique challenges and rules to follow to optimize your healing.

In these pages, you will learn to separate out the different factors that contribute to chronic wounds to help give you the best possible chance to heal your wound. I will use simple language and easy-to-understand stories to illustrate these critical concepts and leave you with actionable interventions to help you find closure in the wound-healing process. My goals here are to (1) explain what a chronic wound is; (2) highlight the most common types of chronic wounds; and (3) define ways to approach your wound healing.

I. Thinking About Your Wound

A chronic wound is one that fails to progress through the normal stages of healing within an expected time frame. The wound lingers and defies the normal mechanisms that the body uses to repair itself. Typically, simple wounds heal within a relatively short and predictable time frame, but chronic wounds can persist for weeks, months, or even years.

The appearance of these wounds can vary widely. Some chronic wounds appear as a trivial opening in the skin that can leave you scratching your head as to how something so simple refuses to heal while other chronic wounds can be large, complex, and so confusing to look at that you wonder how the wound even occurred in the first place. What is common among them is that they are frequently challenging, often frustrating, and sometimes flat-out overwhelming.

Even with the challenges they pose, these wounds are often treatable and often healable. If we understand the causes of these chronic wounds and have the help of a wound care professional, we can often minimize or reverse the factors that cause these wounds and give you the best possible chance for healing.

Chronic wounds often arise from various underlying factors, such as poor blood flow, prolonged inflammation, or a compromised immune response from chronic medical conditions. Conditions like diabetes, arterial or venous insufficiency, pressure injuries, or even surgical complications can contribute to developing a chronic wound. (Don't worry if some of these terms and topics are going over your head right now; we will explain each of these conditions very clearly in short order.)

In the meantime, let's consider the case of a patient of mine named Mr. Trumbull. Mr. T, as I called him, was a middle-aged man who had been battling a persistent diabetic foot ulcer. Mr. T told me he discovered the wound after he noticed a large bright red spot staining the bottom of his sock one evening as he prepared for his nightly shower. He said that on further examination, he noticed a cut with a tiny piece of glass still partially buried below the skin. As we chatted during his initial evaluation, he said, "The weird thing, Doc, is the only time I was around broken glass was about a week ago when I broke a glass in the kitchen and had to sweep it up. I guess I should've put on some slippers, but that's when the glass must've gotten wedged in my foot."

I could tell that this was a difficult concept for Mr. T to wrap his head around, but I told him, "Actually, this kind of thing happens quite commonly with diabetes and the diabetic neuropathy you have."

You see, until that point, Mr. T had not fully faced the extent to which his diabetes had compromised his ability to feel sensation in his feet. It was only the visual sight of the blood-stained sock that alerted him to the wound. The elevated levels of sugar in his blood from his diabetes had damaged the nerves of his legs (diabetic neuropathy) to the point where he was no longer able to feel a cut to his foot, much less the shard of glass that had found a home within the skin and soft tissues of his foot. Because Mr. T was unable to feel the pain that the glass should have caused, it allowed the wound to fester and grow well beyond what it might have been had it been caught earlier. In fact, without that blood-stained sock, the wound very well may have gotten even worse than it was when Mr. T presented it to me.

For months, Mr. T struggled with the slow healing of his diabetic foot ulcer (DFU), leaving him feeling confused and discouraged by the lack of progress. At our appointments, I was able to help Mr. T understand that diabetes is a systemic disease where elevated sugar levels cause damage to cells all throughout his body. We talked about how high sugar levels in the blood affect his normal wound healing in so many different ways.

1. The elevated blood sugar levels in diabetes cause progressive and irreversible injury to the nerves—particularly the nerves that are responsible for sensation in the legs and feet. In medicine, we refer to this phenomenon as "diabetic neuropathy," but in everyday language it simply describes the decreased or abnormal sensation in the skin when it comes to things like light touch, pressure, cuts, and even burns. I explained how his decreased ability to feel his feet put him at risk of developing new and worsening ulcers. For example, if Mr. T could not feel that his shoe did not fit him well, it could lead to excessive rubbing against certain areas of the foot and ankle without his knowledge, which could lead to skin damage, ulcer formation, or worse. In the same way, a lack of sensation could cause him to disregard a small cut or an ingrown toenail he couldn't feel, allowing it to go ignored, fester, and get worse. Similarly, unrealized reinjury and infection due to a lack of sensation can cause complications and setbacks in the healing of known diabetic wounds.

2. The elevated blood sugar level of diabetes scars, narrows, and hardens the blood vessels in a process called "diabetic vasculopathy." It's another fancy medical term that simply refers to a narrowing and hardening of the blood vessels—particularly the vessels in the legs and feet. Think of diabetic vasculopathy as old, bad plumbing. Like corroded pipes in an old house, the flow through these narrow, diseased vessels is weak and slow. We all understand that the circulatory system carries oxygen and nutrients in the blood to all body parts and tissues. However, when blood flow is decreased due to "bad plumbing," the oxygen and nutrient supply no longer efficiently reaches the body parts that need it. Cells, tissues, and body parts

cannot function properly without oxygen. They can become damaged and vulnerable to injury, ultimately predisposing them to wound formation or even tissue death (necrosis). What's worse is that once a wound is formed, without good circulation, the damaged tissues suffer from insufficient oxygen, nutrients, and immune cells—all required for healing. This keeps these diabetic wounds in a dangerous cycle of poor healing. Looking from the patient's perspective, these issues highlight the need for you to take deliberate steps to manage the diabetes and actively treat these wounds.

3 Diabetes also suppresses the immune system. This means that diabetes decreased Mr. T's ability to fight off the "bugs" and bacteria that can cause infection. Mr. T was, therefore, at a higher risk for wound infection than someone without diabetes. Worse still, the immune suppression of diabetes means that identifying a wound infection could be more difficult because all the redness, warmth, and swelling that we would expect to see in a normal infection simply may not be there due to the restricted blood flow. The result, in situations like this, is that identifying an infection is more difficult than in a non-diabetic wound, which can cause delays in treatment, more advanced infections, and setbacks in healing.

While I knew that this was all quite a lot for Mr. T to take in, I was able to explain the concepts and terms in a way that he could relate to and understand. I could see his brow unfurrow and the lines of worry on his face relax as we talked through things during his appointment. Our conversations seemed to lift a fog of confusion that had previously rested over his situation. With the newfound confidence of understanding, Mr. T became more involved in his care. Instead of blindly following instructions from a healthcare provider like me, he was now able to take ownership of his care. He became a more active participant, rather than a passive patient, with more motivation to control the management of his diabetes and ulcer. With this understanding also came a sense of control over his condition and the confidence that he had a say in managing his condition. Mr. T was no longer just along for the ride on his wound care journey; now he could take a more active role in helping his wound heal.

II. Preparing for Your Journey: Approaching Your Wound

A Bird's-Eye View

What can we learn from Mr. Trumbull's story? Well, looking at the big picture, it's important to remember that while complex, Mr. T's story is far from unique. It is actually quite common. In other words, you are not alone. Often, patients feel isolated and alone when it comes to their wounds, but the reality is that there are many, many patients like you, and that there is plenty of help as well.

A significant healthcare challenge, chronic wounds affect tens of millions of people worldwide, and they have become a prevalent health issue in the United States as well. As of 2020, approximately 6.5 million Americans suffer from chronic wounds, and the numbers continue to rise.

Contributing to the rising incidence of chronic wounds is our aging population. Recent decades have seen many advances in and access to healthcare, and data over those same decades shows that we are seeing longer life expectancy, both domestically and worldwide. As life expectancy is increasing, this also means that we are living longer with age-related conditions like weakness, limited mobility, poor nutrition, and thinning skin, which increase our risk of developing chronic wounds. This is not to mention the long list of chronic diseases, like diabetes and circulation problems, which we see most often in older people.

While disease-directed treatments, interventions, and medications do an ever-improving job of managing our diabetes, heart diseases, and the like, they usually don't have quite the same impact on our overall quality of life. The result is often simply that we live in the elderly phase of our lives for a longer period of time and the age-related issues that go along with the advanced years of our lives may contribute to a higher risk of developing a chronic wound or two.

Another very significant factor in the manifestation of chronic wounds is lifestyle choices. Poor diet and nutrition, smoking, and sedentary behavior are endemic in our modern society. We all know intuitively that these choices have a negative effect on our overall health, so it should be no surprise that these same lifestyle choices have very specific negative effects on things like blood flow, the immune system, and even wound healing. It's always in the back of our minds, but it is often overlooked that some of our biggest gains in wound healing can come from the smallest (and admittedly often difficult) decisions of our day-to-day habits and behaviors. I would even go so far as to say that it's this simple truth that led me to write this book. I see it every day, and I want you to realize it too: Small behavior changes and lifestyle decisions can make all the difference between a wound that will heal and one that will not.

Understanding the Wound Care Market

Now, let's talk dollars and cents. Make no mistake about it, the United States' role in the global wound care market is significant. According to The Business Research Company, the American population spent a whopping $12.1 billion on the wound care market in 2021. That was almost half of the global pie, which is projected to grow from $26.2 billion in 2021 to $38.8 billion in 2026 worldwide.

So why is the US wound care market so huge? Well, the reasons are the same as I highlighted before. First, our population is getting older, and as we age, we tend to need more wound care supplies and services, which drives the demand for wound care products. Second, healthcare costs are on the rise across the board, and treating wounds can be expensive. And third, an increase in the number and complexity of wound infections delay wound healing further pushes up the cost of treatment due to the need for more advanced and more expensive antimicrobial products.

More than half of the cost of long-term wound care occurs in hospitals and nursing homes for the various surgeries, interventions, procedures, and treatments performed in these settings. And despite medical advancements, it is the wound dressings—the gauze, bandages, creams, ointments, and tape—that still account for more than half of wound care's market share dollars.

In a nutshell, the US is by far the biggest player in the wound care landscape, driven by factors like our aging population, rising healthcare costs, and evermore complicated infection issues. Wound dressings constitute the highest cost in wound care, while hospitals, nursing homes, and increasingly the home health setting are key places where these products are used.

Chronic Wounds: Not Your Typical Wound

What sets chronic wounds apart from regular wounds is the complex way in which they heal. These wounds often extend through the skin into deeper tissues like muscle, fat, and even bone. Chronic wounds are often characterized by their poor healing progression. Healing is often slow or delayed due to a lack of *inflammation*. We all know what it's like to have a sore and swollen toe after stubbing it on a piece of furniture. Well, that redness, throbbing, and swelling is inflammation. It is the product of all the biological processes that help to protect the wounded area from further injury and help it to heal. Inflammation increases circulation to a wounded area, bringing enriching blood and oxygen. This explains the swelling and increased warmth you feel in inflamed tissues.

Also, in the cascade of events of inflammation is the process of *angiogenesis*, by which new blood vessels grow inside a wound. These new blood vessels of angiogenesis are what bring blood, oxygen, and nutrients to the middle of a wound bed. Equally important in the healing process is the formation of new *granulation tissue*–that all-important combination of new cells and protein that fills the empty space of an open, chronic wound. Finally, wound healing is "capped off" by *epithelialization*, where a layer of epithelial tissue (skin tissue) grows over the top of the wound's bed of granulation tissue to complete the healing process.

I like to think of the healing wound as similar to working on a construction site. Now, imagine a construction site where the job is, say, to create a parking lot. But, instead of workers pouring cement over open ground, healthy cells in a wound bed work together to lay down a cushiony bed of granulation tissue. Angiogenesis creates the roadways that carry the materials needed for healing into the construction site. Healthy cells within the wound bed are the workers laying down the granulation tissue to fill the wound bed. Obviously, the more workers there are at the construction site, the faster the job gets done. Granulation tissue fills in the wound from the bottom to the top, and then epithelialization is that final layer of asphalt that covers everything to protect all the work that was done below. By thinking about wounds and wound healing in terms we can all relate to, it becomes so much easier to understand the basics of wound healing.

On the flip side, there are any number of issues that can stall this well-coordinated healing process. Large amounts of drainage from the open wound, necrotic (dead) tissue in the wound bed, and infection can upend, complicate, and even completely stop wound healing. What's worse is that issues like these can prevent wound healing, make a wound bed less than healthy, and can even make a wound larger. If there are too many negative factors in and around the wound, the deck quickly gets stacked against us, wound healing stalls, and we're left with a wound that will not heal. So, let's look at the tools and information needed to tip the scales of wound healing back in our favor.

Keeping It in Perspective

All of the terminology, physiology, and treatment options can get over-whelming very quickly when it comes to chronic wound healing. There was a time years ago when I, too, had to learn all of this for the first time, so I know how the abundance of information can feel like drinking water from a fire hydrant. Trust me though, this is something you can manage. And I am here to help guide you along the way.

In this book, I'll describe various clinical scenarios to help paint clear pictures of what wounds look like and how you should approach healing them. I'll break down relevant issues in easy-to-understand language. We'll use relatable concepts, and I'll stick to just the information you need to know. In addition to describing all the issues related to wound healing, I have compiled a set of appendices at the end of this book as a quick reference for information that will surely help answer your questions along the way: tools like a glossary of common terms used in wound care, common wound care dressings and products, and much more.

The management of chronic wounds has advanced significantly over the years, offering various treatment options and strategies to promote healing. Your doctor or wound care clinician is best equipped to determine how to leverage these innovative therapies and decide on a treatment plan custom-ized to meet your specific needs. We will not be discussing the ins and outs of various treatment options here (but do use the helpful appendices at the end of this book for more information on specific dressings and products that your wound care provider may decide to use). Instead, we'll focus on embracing a high-level but comprehensive approach to wound care. This includes addressing the underlying causes and optimizing wound bed conditions to empower you and supercharge your healing process.

Remember, your body knows how to repair and heal itself. Usually, it is the underlying medical conditions, the advanced age, the limited mobility, the poor nutrition, etc., that get in the way of the regular healing process. Our first job is to identify the factors standing in the way of wound healing in your individual case and then address them one by one. We will be able to modify some issues, such as nutrition and patient poisoning, while other issues, like decreased mobility, may not be something we can change directly. The goal here is to control what we can to create an environment within the wound bed that best supports and hopefully accelerates the ordered steps of wound healing that your body is designed to perform.

Wounds are like individuals: Each one is unique. Some are cooperative, while others are very, very stubborn. They come in different shapes, sizes, and appearances. They even vary in the locations where they exist. However, just like people, for all their differences, every single one has similar basic needs. Of course, there are nuances to every wound. Your doctor or wound care provider will help you navigate these nuances, tailor your treatment plan, and use all the recent advancements in wound care at his disposal.

Here, I simply want you to understand the basic medical, physical, and environmental issues that underlie your wound. We will create a foundation of understanding that will be the basis for your wound healing success. As with anything, knowledge is power. So, take a deep breath, calm your nerves, and rest assured that the information in the pages ahead will contain the keys to success that will empower you along your path to healing.

III. Understanding Your Wound

To begin managing chronic wounds, it is important to understand exactly what we are dealing with. I mean, if you are trying to fix a problem—any problem—doesn't it make sense to understand what caused the problem in the first place? With chronic wounds, we first need to know what types of wounds there are. It also helps to know which types of wounds occur on which body parts. Most importantly, though, we must understand the medical issues, anatomic problems, and lifestyle choices that put us at risk for developing a particular kind of wound in the first place. This is especially important because it's often the case that the very same risk factors that cause these wounds are also the reason why chronic wounds linger longer than they should. In the sections ahead, we will delve into all the particulars of the different wound types, the factors that contribute to their chronic nature, and strategies for how to approach and heal them.

Skin Protection

Before we dive in, it's worth taking a little bit of time to discuss the skin and soft tissues (the body's protective and cushiony layers), especially since the skin is usually where we see the first evidence of tissue injury and wounds.

The skin is your body's largest organ, covering your entire external surface and acting as a protective barrier between you and the outside world. It has three main layers:

1. The epidermis is the outermost layer, protecting you from water loss, sunlight, and germs.

2 The dermis lies beneath the epidermis and provides support to your skin. This is where the blood vessels, nerves, hair follicles, and glands of the skin live.

3 The deepest layer is known as the subcutaneous layer. Subcutaneous tissue is made up of fat cells called "adipocytes," as well as connective tissue and blood vessels. Together, the tissues of the subcutaneous layer help with insulation, energy storage, and cushioning, providing protection to the underlying structures such as muscles, bones, and organs.

Your skin has many important functions. It protects you from harmful substances like germs and chemicals and also helps regulate your body temperature. It has receptors on its surface that allow you to feel sensations such as light touch, pressure, pain, and temperature. Additionally, your skin plays a role in absorbing certain substances and excreting waste products.

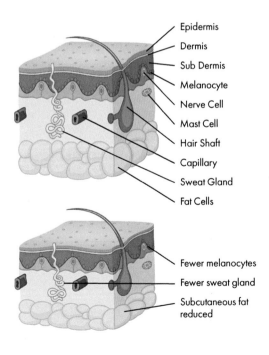

Epidermis
Dermis
Sub Dermis
Melanocyte
Nerve Cell
Mast Cell
Hair Shaft
Capillary
Sweat Gland
Fat Cells

Fewer melanocytes
Fewer sweat gland
Subcutaneous fat reduced

Skin and Skin Aging

More than wrinkles and age spots, profound changes occur to skin with aging that impair wound healing. As the skin's collagen and elastin fibers diminish with age, there is a loss of elasticity and firmness. The skin becomes thinner and more fragile, making it prone to bruising and damage. As skin ages, it requires increased care and attention to maintain its health and integrity.

Understanding the structure and function of the skin is important in discussing chronic wounds and wound care. It follows, then, that a cornerstone of wound care and prevention is diligent skin care. Keeping the skin clean, hydrated, and moisturized is critical to supporting skin health. Simple skincare techniques—cleansing, hydrating, and moisturizing—go far in preventing new wounds and improving the skin quality around open wounds to allow them to heal well. Here is how:

- Regular bathing clears the skin of dead cells, dirt, and debris that can break down the epidermal layer.

- Drinking water to stay well hydrated gives the skin volume, strength, suppleness, and pliability.

- Regular use of your favorite moisturizer, particularly after you bathe, helps trap moisture against the skin, keeping it hydrated, healthy, and happy. You have to remember that even small cracks caused by dryness of the skin and damage can set the stage for cellulitis, infection, and wound formation. This is why I cannot stress enough the importance of using a skin moisturizer at least once a day to help keep your body's largest organ, the skin, functioning as it should.

So, now that we have this background information, let's go deeper into chronic wounds and how we can manage them effectively for closure. Remember, this summary provides a brief overview of the skin's structure and function to set the stage for a more in-depth discussion with your healthcare provider regarding chronic wounds and wound care.

Pressure Wounds

Let's start by discussing one of the more ominous wound types associated with mobility, aging, and severe illness: pressure injury (sometimes called "bedsores" or "pressure ulcers"). How do pressure injury wounds occur, and are there factors that put an individual at risk of developing them?

Remember, your skin is that strong yet cushiony layer of tissue protecting the underlying tissues, bones, and organs. When excessive pressure is applied to a specific area for too long, it can disrupt the blood flow to the skin, leading to skin damage and pressure injury. As an example, let's imagine you are sitting on a hard bench, engrossed in a sporting event or captivating movie. What you are watching is so good that you lose track of time and hardly take notice of anything else going on. As things come to an end, you get up and notice soreness in a couple of areas on your rear end, maybe even with an associated red mark or two. Well, that soreness and redness is a pressure injury in its mildest form. This is the effect of all your body weight resting on one or two of your gluteal bones for too long. The skin and subcutaneous tissue of your buttocks, unfortunately, get caught between the weight of your body and the hard bench below. Blood vessels leading to the area get crushed, cutting off blood flow to the skin and subcutaneous tissue. At first, it causes pain, and then, as time goes by, more and more tissue damage at the very spot where pressure is applied. By sitting too long without moving, any of us can eventually develop a pressure sore on our buttocks.

To show you how it tends to work with actual pressure wound patients, let me tell you about a couple of people whom I have treated. First, there was Mr. Johnson. Mr. Johnson spent most of his day confined to a wheelchair. At the advanced age of 87, general body weakness severely limited his mobility. He could not stand for more than a few seconds at a time and even had difficulty with shifting his weight and changing positions in his wheelchair. Another patient, Mrs. Oliver, had been bedridden for several weeks due to an illness when I met her. Because she did not understand the consequences of not regularly moving her body (even when in bed), Mrs. Oliver found her most comfortable position in that bed and stayed there, often for extended periods of time. Both patients were at high risk for pressure injury, which they unfortunately developed.

What causes these pressure injuries? In a word, *"pressure."* We all may experience some measure of pressure injury on a regular basis, but in able-bodied folks, feedback loops in the brain subconsciously tell us when it's time to get out of our bed or chair to relieve the pressure and keep us from these kinds of pressure injuries. The feedback loops, where our body tells our brain to do something, and we do it without even thinking (kind of like a reflex), is why we find the need to shift our weight from time to time if we have been sitting too long–say like in a chair when sitting at a desk or on a long car ride. Those little shifts we barely acknowledge are our bodies protecting themselves from pressure injuries. On the other hand, with weakness or impaired mobility–where our bodies cannot move easily–these feedback loops gradually get ignored over time, leading to sustained pressure that can cause tissue damage and deep wounds. Limited mobility can occur for a variety of reasons, including muscle weakness, paralysis, recent surgery, illness, or prolonged bed rest.

Pressure injuries commonly occur at places where body weight is focused on a small area, such as the heels, hips, sacrum (lower back), shoulders, and elbows. We call these parts of the body "pressure points." Maybe you remember that equation from school that says $P = F/A$. If you are scratching your head right now, don't worry. Physics class was quite a while ago for most of us, but $P = F/A$ is the equation that states [P]ressure equals [F]orce divided by [A]rea.

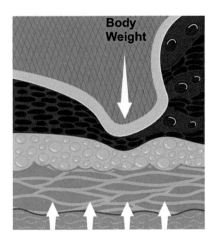

Understanding Pressure Points

Pressure is greatest when distributed over small areas. When body weight is focused on small bony areas like the heel or the tailbone the skin, fat, and muscle in the area are caught between the bone and the surface the body is on. The tissues are deformed and the blood vessels leading to these areas are pressed closed. Under the body's weight, tissues in bony areas like this can become injured and lack the blood supply to help the tissues recover and heal.

To bring that equation to life, imagine you're pushing your open hand down on the surface of a table. Go ahead, push hard. No problem, right? You might even be able to support much of your body weight on that hand. That is because the force is spread over a large surface area between the palm of your hand and the table, reducing the pressure. But press your index finger against a corner of that same table. Well, now, that's a different story, isn't it? The pressure suddenly becomes very intense, doesn't it? It's because all that force is now focused on a very small area, causing the pressure (and pain) to shoot up intensely. This focused, intense pressure is precisely why pressure ulcers tend to occur in areas where the body weight is concentrated on small, bony prominences known as pressure points. These pressure points are the areas we need to know and protect to help prevent and treat pressure injuries.

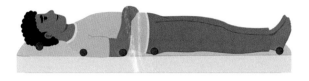

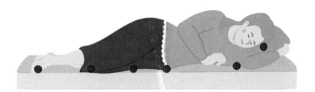

Pressure Point Locations

- Back of Head
- Shoulders
- Elbows
- Sacrum (tailbone)
- Hips
- Buttocks
- Knees
- Ankles
- Heels

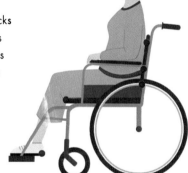

Another important concept in the development of pressure injuries is "shear." Shear occurs when there is a combination of pressure and friction or when the skin moves in one direction while the underlying tissues move in the opposite direction. It is like when you drag a heavy object across the floor, and it causes a rug burn. Shear forces can further damage already vulnerable skin and contribute to the development of pressure injuries.

Stages of Pressure Injury

The common thread of pressure injury wounds is sustained or prolonged pressure on the skin and underlying tissues from an underlying surface. Pressure injuries develop when an individual remains immobile for an extended period, causing restricted blood flow to specific areas of the body. The mainstay of both prevention and treatment of pressure injuries is the same - regular repositioning, good skincare, and the use of appropriate support surfaces to help off-load vulnerable pressure points on the body.

Stage 1 - Non-Blanchable Skin Redness

Redness of the skin over a pressure point that does not go away when the red area is touched.

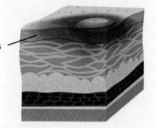

Epidermis

Stage 2 - Broken / Peeled Skin

Tissue damage over a pressure point that goes into the skin, but not through the skin.

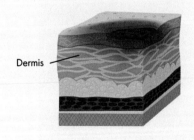

Dermis

Note: The descriptions of pressure injury below may be more noticeable in fair-skinned individuals and the detection of the early stage pressure injury may be more subtle in people with darker skin.

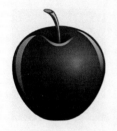

Stage 1 - Non-Blanchable Skin Redness
When you press on the healthy skin of the palm of your hand it temporarily lightens in color. This is called 'blanching'. In contrast, a stage 1 pressure injury shows redness that doesn't fade (or 'blanch') when pressed. Imagine pressing the skin of a red apple - the color stays the same. Stage 1 skin, like the apple peel, has a fixed red color but the skin isn't broken.

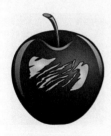

Stage 2 - Broken / Peeled Skin
If you keep pressing or rubbing on the injured area of an apple, the skin eventually breaks. This is similar to a stage 2 pressure injury. Part of the top layers of skin (peel) are damaged or rubbed off, but it doesn't go deep.

Stage 3 - Damage into Flesh

Tissue damage overlying a pressure point that goes through the skin and into the fat below the skin (subcutaneous tissue), but there is no exposed muscle, tendon or bone within the wound.

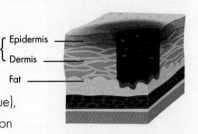

Skin { Epidermis
Dermis

Fat

Stage 4 - Exposed Anatomic Structures

Tissue damage overlying a pressure point that goes through the skin, subcutaneous tissue down to muscle, tendon or bone.

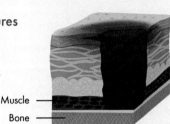

Muscle

Bone

Deep Tissue Pressure Injury - Deep Bruise

Injury to the tissue beneath the skin even while the skin is intact. Deep Tissue Pressure Injury appears as deeply bruised skin to the eye and may feel 'mushy' to the touch.

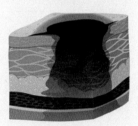

Unstageable Pressure Injury - Necrotic Tissue Present

A wound where the stage can not be determined because necrotic (dead) tissue, like slough or eschar, sits in the middle of the wound hiding its true depth.

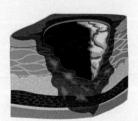

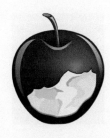

Stage 3 - Damage into Flesh

Take a bite out of the apple, but not all the way to the core. This represents a stage 3 pressure injury. There's a noticeable bite (wound) that goes through the peel (skin) and deeper into the apple (fatty tissue), but it doesn't reach the core (muscle or bone).

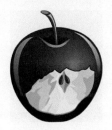

Stage 4 - Exposed Anatomic Structures

If you bite deeper into the apple, reaching the core (muscle or bone), that's like a stage 4 pressure injury. The bite (wound) is severe, exposing deeper tissues like muscle or bone, similar to the core of the apple.

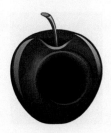

Deep Tissue Pressure Injury - Deep Bruise

Imagine a bruised apple. In addition to discoloration of the peel (skin), there is damage to the inner flesh as well. Damage occurs to the skin and underlying flesh, without any visible breaks in the skin itself.

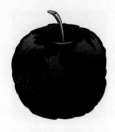

Unstageable Pressure Injury - Necrotic Tissue Present

Imagine an apple that has sat out for too long. The apple may be brown and mushy in some spots or hard and dried-out in others. There is injury, but the dead areas on the surface do not make it possible to assess (or stage) the damage below.

So, let's summarize what we have learned here. First, these are the risk factors for pressure injuries:

- Limited mobility or immobility

- Prolonged pressure on small, bony areas

- Poor nutrition and hydration

- Age-related changes in the skin

- Chronic illnesses that affect blood flow and tissue health

Second, to prevent and treat pressure injuries, it's important to:

- Frequently reposition or shift your body weight every couple of hours

- Use specialized cushions or pillows to redistribute and alleviate pressure

- Maintain good nutrition and hydration to support healthy skin

- Regularly inspect your skin for any signs of redness, warmth, or breakdown

- Maintain good hygiene and keep the skin clean and dry

- Use gentle moisturizers to keep the skin hydrated and supple

- Avoid excessive friction or shear on the skin by using body positioners as well as proper lifting and transferring techniques for physically limited individuals

There, that's it. Now you have a strong fundamental grasp of pressure injury wounds and why they happen. That wasn't too painful, right? You also have a relatively simple set of strategies that, along with appropriate medical care, will significantly increase your chances of healing your pressure injury wound, reduce the risk of developing new pressure injuries, and help you to maintain your overall skin health.

Diabetic Wounds

Now, let's dive into how and why the ominous diabetic wounds occur. Sugar diabetes, or just diabetes, is that awful condition where someone we know has lost a toe or a foot because of ulcers and/or infection. For some people, uncontrolled diabetes leads to heart disease or loss of vision, while for others, diabetes damages the kidneys to the point where patients need lifelong dialysis. We've all heard the horror stories; we know them well. So then, if we know the consequences, why do we ever let the consequences of diabetes get to such a point?

Well, at least part of it is because high blood sugar levels cause slow, silent damage that goes largely unnoticed until it's often too late. There's often no pain, no swelling, and no discomfort associated with elevated sugar levels as it does its damage. What's more is that historically, it has been difficult for diabetic patients to test their blood sugar levels as they should, day-to-day and hour by hour. On top of all of this, the medication regimens for diabetes can be challenging to administer. Because there are no warning signs, no immediate consequences, and no easy ways to manage diabetes, the tissue damage of diabetes often occurs in silence, day by day, from the inside of the body out. This is typically why by the time the tissue damage of diabetes presents itself, the damage is already done: Vision has been lost; damage to the heart has occurred; or deep, complicated infections have developed.

While the well-known stories of diabetes damaging the eyes, heart, kidneys, and toes suggest that diabetes affects only certain body parts, it is important to remember that diabetes is a systemic disease. This means the elevated sugar levels of diabetes affect nearly all tissues throughout the entire body. If you think about it, it kind of makes sense. The elevated sugars are carried in the circulating blood, and since the blood circulates everywhere to provide oxygen and nutrients to all cells, then all those cells are also exposed to the elevated sugar levels.

What is more, diabetes is a progressive disease, so without intervention to lower the average sugar level, the disease will continue to get worse until it causes cellular injury, disability, organ failure, or even tissue death. Diabetes is silent in its nature and progressive in the damage it causes. It's scary when you know; however, the problem is that many patients don't know. Either they don't see their doctor regularly and don't know they have diabetes, they don't know how dangerous it will be to ignore the diagnosis, or they don't know how to overcome the many challenges of following and treating the disease. Since the silent damage of diabetes largely stays out of sight, the urgency to control one's diabetes often stays out of mind for many diabetics and prediabetics.

One of the main reasons why diabetes is able to do such widespread damage is because it causes injury to the small blood vessels and tiny capillaries of the body. These tiny, delicate blood vessels are the place where oxygen in the blood hops out of the bloodstream and is delivered to the organs and tissues of your body. We call it the microvasculature—"micro" for small + "vasculature" for blood vessels. Organs like your heart, lungs, kidneys, and skin then use the oxygen and nutrients from the blood to function properly. However, in diabetes, the high levels of sugar in the blood cause scarring, narrowing, and hardening of the microvasculature, leading to irreversible damage to these delicate blood vessels. All that damage affects future blood flow and limits the delivery of oxygen to the end organs. Without a healthy and properly functioning microvasculature, oxygen simply cannot make it to the organs that need it, and the organs themselves become damaged as well.

If this all sounds a bit abstract so far, don't worry. Let's paint a picture that should help make this concept stick a little better. Think of the blood vessels as roads that transport blood throughout the body. The large blood vessels in your body, such as arteries and veins, are like highways and turnpikes, efficiently carrying blood over long distances and quickly getting oxygen and nutrients to different regions of the body. However, the smaller blood vessels and capillaries (microvasculature) are like the streets in your city or town, delivering blood and oxygen to all the individual tissues and organs that need them—kind of like an Uber driver delivering food to your home when you're hungry.

Now imagine driving through your town, but the normal roadways are all damaged and detoured. Your once wide, open city streets are more like a congested downtown where cars move slowly and struggle to reach their destination. In a sense, this is what happens in diabetes. While congestion in the streets may mean your Uber dinner delivery is delayed, when it happens in the microvasculature, oxygen and nutrients don't get to the tissues that need them in time. Without enough oxygen, the cells and organs cannot function well, leading to end organ damage that only gets worse with time. Organs everywhere can be affected in this way, including the eyes, kidneys, heart, and more. This is why controlling your blood sugar levels is critical in diabetes management. Controlling your blood sugar is the single best way we have to limit the progression of end-organ damage and other complications of diabetes. When your blood sugar is well managed, it reduces the scarring and narrowing of the microvasculature and helps protect and preserve the tissues.

In addition to vascular injury and end-organ damage, nerve damage (also known as "neuropathy") is a common complication of diabetes. When your nerves are affected, you may experience reduced or altered sensation in certain areas like your legs and feet. This lack of sensation makes it harder to detect injuries like cuts or blisters, as was the case with Mr. Trumbull, whom I discussed earlier.

If we know what diabetic vascular disease is and we know what diabetic neuropathy is, then we understand the two major factors that give rise to diabetic ulcers. When microvascular injury and nerve damage combine, areas like the feet become particularly vulnerable to ulcer formation for

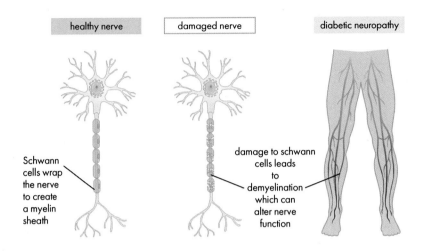

healthy nerve | damaged nerve | diabetic neuropathy

Schwann cells wrap the nerve to create a myelin sheath

damage to schwann cells leads to demyelination which can alter nerve function

Understanding Diabetic Neuropathy

The elevated blood sugar levels of diabetes affect systems throughout the body. In the nervous system, high sugars can lead to the process where there is damage to or loss of the protective myelin sheath that covers, protects, and insulates nerve fibers (demyelination). In the body, myelin is like the rubber insulation around an electrical wire. When demyelination occurs nerves may not work correctly leading to symptoms such as numbness, tingling, and weakness, particularly in the extremities.

diabetics. Unlike someone who does not have nerve damage, a diabetic may not feel a small cut or new blister forming due to their reduced ability to feel their feet. On top of this, that small injury will often fail to heal properly due to the poor circulation caused by the diabetic vascular disease we discussed above. It is this combination of conditions that leads to the deterioration and downward spiral of diabetic ulcers. A small injury goes ignored or untreated. It lingers. The wound then gets further injured due to everyday wear and tear from normal activities. The wound slowly gets bigger with time; all the while, the diabetic patient feels little to no discomfort from any of it. Inevitably, infection develops in the wound, further complicating things. It all creates a recipe for disaster.

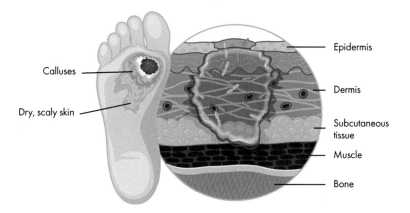

Calluses

Dry, scaly skin

Epidermis

Dermis

Subcutaneous tissue

Muscle

Bone

Diabetic Ulcers

Diabetic ulcers are notoriously complex and challenging to heal for several reasons. First, diabetes can affect the blood vessels decreasing blood flow, oxygen, and nutrients to the wound site. Secondly, diabetic neuropathy can cause reduced sensation in the affected area, making patients less aware of developing problems with the wound. Lastly, the high blood sugars of diabetes can affect the immune system in a few ways: (1) by reducing the body's ability to fight off bacteria and prevent wound infections and (2) by promoting inflammation that limits the formation of new blood vessels to the wound. All of these challenges make diabetic ulcers particularly difficult to heal.

There are several risk factors for the development of diabetic ulcers. People who have had diabetes for a long time or who have poorly controlled blood sugar levels are at the highest risk. Risk factors include:

- Diabetic neuropathy (nerve damage) and reduced sensation in the feet

- Foot deformities, such as bunions and hammertoes, which can lead to new pressure points on the feet

- Smoking, which impairs blood flow and delays wound healing

- Poor foot care and hygiene

- Wearing ill-fitting shoes that cause pressure on certain areas of the feet

Open diabetic ulcers are also at risk for complications such as infections, which can be quite severe. However, with proper care and awareness, they can often be effectively treated or prevented. For example, checking your feet regularly for cuts, blisters, or injuries—especially if you are experiencing reduced sensation—is essential.

Here are some other practical strategies for preventing diabetic ulcers and managing diabetic foot health:

- Control blood sugar levels within the target range through diet, exercise, and medications as prescribed by your healthcare provider.

- Regularly inspect your feet for any cuts, blisters, or injuries, especially if you have reduced sensation.

- Keep your feet clean and dry, and moisturize them to prevent cracks and dryness.

- Wear well-fitting shoes and consider using custom orthotic inserts to reduce pressure on specific areas.

- Avoid smoking as it can impair blood flow and hinder wound healing.

- Work closely with your healthcare provider to manage your diabetes and foot health.

Remember, diabetic wounds are a consequence of the severity and duration of your diabetes. By being proactive and taking care of your overall health, you can significantly reduce the risk of diabetic ulcers as well as their potential complications.

Arterial Wounds

To understand peripheral arterial disease (PAD) and arterial ulcers, let's go back to our analogy of the circulatory system as streets and highways. We said to think of the large blood vessels in your body like highways and turnpikes, efficiently carrying blood over long distances to different regions of the body while the smaller blood vessels and capillaries are like the streets of your city or town, delivering blood and oxygen to all the tissues and organs that need them. In the case of arterial wounds, we are talking about the large blood vessels in your body or the "highways." These highway-like blood vessels are long and relatively wide, carrying the blood over long distances from your heart to different parts of your body, including all the way down to the toes.

Unfortunately, just like on a highway, traffic jams can occur. And—as you know—when they do, they bring everything to a slow, slow crawl. In the case of PAD, a condition called "atherosclerosis" creates the equivalent of a traffic jam on the blood vessel superhighway. Atherosclerosis refers to the buildup of plaque inside the walls of the blood vessels, which can narrow a four-lane highway of a blood vessel to just one or two slow lanes of through traffic. Just like bumper-to-bumper traffic, when blockages occur, blood moves sluggishly rather than smoothly and efficiently. Not only this, but this type of blood vessel narrowing can occur in multiple locations along the blood vessel super-highway—one accident after another on the highway. The result of blood vessel narrowing and blockages is decreased blood flow to the tissues that follow these lesions. This can lead to a number of symptoms and complications.

It's important to note here that PAD shares similarities with coronary artery disease (CAD), or "heart disease." While PAD involves narrowing and blockages in the blood vessels that lead to the legs and feet, CAD similarly affects the blood vessels supplying the heart. Both conditions involve atherosclerosis and poor blood flow, just on different "highways" of the body.

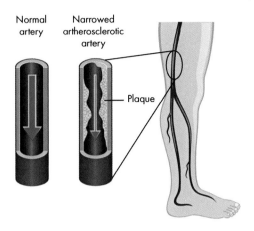

Understanding PAD

Peripheral arterial disease (or narrowing of the arteries) is caused by the continuous accumulation of fatty deposits within the wall of the arteries of the leg which progressively narrows the size of the artery and limits blood flow. Reduced blood flow can lead to pain, ulcers, gangrene, and tissue loss. In Arterial disease, it is important to modify any and all lifestyle issues that may be contributing to the arterial disease like obesity, smoking, hyperlipidemia, diabetes, hypertension, and a sedentary lifestyle.

Arterial ulcers often develop on the legs or feet due to reduced blood flow, and they are particularly challenging to heal. In PAD, lesions in the blood vessels limit blood flow to healthy-appearing tissue, leaving them more susceptible than usual. PAD lesions can even completely block the delivery of blood to ulcers and injured tissues, which can severely slow down or even prevent wound healing from occurring at all. Wounds can be deep and painful with a pale, "punched-out" appearance. In extreme cases, the tissue can be completely dry, hard, dark, and even necrotic from the lack of blood flow to the area.

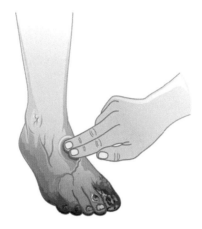

Arterial Injury

In peripheral arterial disease (PAD) there are blockages within the arteries of the limbs, most commonly the legs and feet. This condition often presents with symptoms such as cramping, pain, or discomfort in the legs during physical activity due to limited blood flow. As PAD progresses, it can lead to more severe symptoms like leg pain at rest, bluish or pale discoloration of the skin of the legs, and non-healing ulcers on the feet or toes. Early diagnosis is crucial to preventing the complications of PAD and improving the quality of life.

Certain factors can speed up the progression of PAD, such as smoking, high blood pressure, high cholesterol, and diabetes. On the other hand, there are behaviors that can help alleviate the symptoms and manage PAD. For example, regular exercise can improve circulation and strengthen the muscles. It's important to find a balance between activity and rest, gradually increasing your exercise tolerance.

In managing the signs and symptoms of PAD, here are some practical strategies you can follow:

- Quit smoking: Smoking damages the blood vessels and worsens **PAD**. Quitting smoking can significantly improve blood flow and your overall health.

- Manage underlying medical conditions: Controlling blood pressure, cholesterol, and blood sugar levels is crucial in managing **PAD** and preventing further complications.

- Maintain a healthy lifestyle: Eat a well-balanced diet that is rich in fruits, vegetables, and whole grains. This keeps your blood vessels healthy and reduces the risk of further arterial damage.

- Take care of your feet: Check your feet regularly for any sores, cuts, or blisters. Keep them clean and moisturized. Proper foot care can help prevent the development of arterial ulcers.

- Seek medical care: Regular visits to your healthcare provider are essential for monitoring your condition and adjusting medications as needed.

Arterial ulcers, resulting from reduced blood flow and arterial injury, can be challenging to heal. The lack of proper blood supply makes it difficult for wounds to receive the necessary nutrients and oxygen for healing. Factors like poor circulation, impaired immune response, and underlying health conditions can further complicate the healing process. To summarize, here is a list of risk factors that exacerbate **PAD** and arterial wounds:

- Smoking

- High blood pressure

- High cholesterol levels

- Diabetes

- Obesity

- A low-activity, sedentary lifestyle

Therefore, here are some best practices for treating and managing PAD:

- Quit smoking

- Control blood pressure, cholesterol, and diabetes

- Maintain a healthy lifestyle with regular exercise and a balanced diet

- Practice good foot care and hygiene

- Regularly visit your healthcare provider to monitor and make adjustments to your treatment plan

Remember, by taking control of your health and following the strategies listed above, you can effectively manage your PAD and improve your overall well-being.

Venous Ulcers

Now that we've explained arterial circulation, which carries blood from the heart out to the tissues and organs, let's take a look at venous circulation, which brings blood from the tissues back to the heart. To do this, let's imagine a roller coaster. Arterial circulation is like that effortless part of the ride where the coaster is racing downhill, and the blood is propelled by the pumping action of the heart, flowing quickly through arteries to deliver oxygen and nutrients to the tissues.

The venous circulation, on the other hand, is like the steady uphill climb that takes the roller coaster up the hill before it starts its descent. It's a slow, coordinated process like the ratcheting "click, click, click" of gears pulling the coaster slowly up its incline. Like the coaster, the climb of blood through the venous system back to the heart is effortful and slow. To facilitate this uphill journey, instead of gears, the veins use small, one-way valves that open to allow blood to flow toward the heart and then close to prevent backward flow (also known as "venous reflux"). Think of these valves like the turnstile gates at the amusement park. The gate turns easily to let you walk through in one direction but locks behind you so you don't go backward the wrong way. Just like turnstile gates, the valves in the veins keep blood moving forward in the right direction back to the heart.

In the case of venous disease, however, the valves become damaged, and the valves that were only supposed to open one way now can swing freely back and forth. Instead of the venous blood moving in only one direction toward the heart, some blood sloshes backward (refluxes) through the broken valve, causing a backup of blood in the veins. The reflux causes blood to pool within the veins, creating a column of increasing pressure within them. As the old saying goes, "pressure bursts pipes," and all that pressure from pooling blood in the veins can cause them to stretch, crack, and even leak.

As a patient, you might see these effects first as swollen varicose veins under the skin or maybe even as swelling (or edema) of the entire leg. The high blood pressure within the veins damages the veins and kicks off a whole cascade of inflammatory changes that we know as venous stasis disease (or venous insufficiency). The changes to the skin and soft tissue that follow can cause a whole host of problems, including skin inflammation, skin blistering, skin drainage, and tissue ulceration.

Edema, or tissue swelling, occurs when the increased pressure in the veins causes the veins to leak fluid, like damaged pipes. When the veins leak, the extra fluid collects within the subcutaneous tissues of the legs. The fluid buildup then stretches the skin, which can lead to irritation and inflammation of the skin, known as stasis dermatitis. Because the skin is inflamed, broken, and/or damaged, it also becomes more susceptible to things like infections, cellulitis, and further skin damage. On top of this, as edema builds, so too does the stretching and injury to the skin, which leads to

Normal vein
with working
valves

Abnormal,
dilated vein with
Incompetent Valves

Varicose
veins

Understanding Vein Valve Dysfunction

Vein valve dysfunction is when the one-way valves in the veins of
the legs fail to function properly to move blood back to the heart.
When they malfunction blood can pool in the veins, leading to
varicose veins, leg swelling, leg pain, skin changes, and ulceration.
This condition can be caused by factors like genetics, prolonged
standing or sitting, trauma, obesity, and aging. Venous disease
like this must be managed with lifestyle changes - leg elevation,
compression stockings, walking and, in some cases, medical
procedures to repair or replace the faulty valves.

progressive skin breakdown, skin openings, weeping of edema fluid and,
ultimately, open venous ulcers.

As you probably noticed by now, the issue of "fluid" keeps coming up in
regard to these venous wounds—pressure from too much fluid in the veins,
fluid accumulation in the legs, and fluid leakage from weeping skin. This is
because, in venous disease, the extra fluid is the central factor in the skin
injury and tissue breakdown associated with these wounds.

Wound Drainage

Now is probably a good time to take a moment to briefly discuss the effects of fluid on wound healing, venous wounds, and otherwise. Think back to the last time you hopped out of the bathtub or a swimming pool after a long soak. Remember how your hands looked, all pruned and waterlogged? You might have even rubbed your hands and fingers together, only to see some of that top skin layer peel right off. Kind of gross, I know, but it perfectly illustrates the extent to which excess moisture can affect skin and soft tissues. In wound care, we call it "tissue maceration." Maceration is like that pruning effect on your hands and fingers, but on steroids.

When the skin around a wound becomes oversaturated with moisture, just like your fingers in the pool, the skin can become soft, soggy, and weak. This can happen if a wound is making too

DESCRIPTION	QUALITIES	SIGNIFICANCE
Serous	Clear or light yellow Thin, watery liquid	Normal healing response
Serosanguinous	Clear of slightly cloudy Pink or light red color Thin, watery liquid	Normal healing response
Sanguineous	Bright red color Bloody Thicker than serous fluid	Hemorrhage Bleeding may be trivial or significant
Purulent	Pus - a creamy or milky discharge Thick and opaque Can be yellow, tan, greenish Can have a foul odor	Purulent fluid is a sign of infection. Pus may contain infectious bacteria or viruses

much fluid, a bandage doesn't allow the skin to breathe properly, or if there's excessive edema fluid (like with venous disease) below the wound bed looking for a way out. This is a problem because, just like your wrinkly fingers, macerated skin around the wound becomes fragile and more susceptible to breakdown and infection. It loses its natural strength and protective barrier function, making it harder to heal the wound effectively. The same can be said for subcutaneous and soft tissues. When muscle and fat are exposed to too much moisture, they, too, can break down and slough away, making your wound even larger and more challenging to heal.

So, as a principle, whether we are talking about venous wounds or any other type of chronic wound, we always want to make sure to keep the skin surrounding a wound clean and dry, the same way you would dry off your hands after a bath or swim. We try to choose dressings and bandages that help absorb excessive moisture while also allowing the skin to breathe. By controlling moisture balance, we can avoid skin maceration and give the wound the best chance to heal smoothly.

On the other hand, at least some moisture is needed in the wound bed for the wound to heal. Good moisture balance within the wound bed keeps new cells and healing tissues happy and allows normal biological processes to occur. For my own wound care patients, I generally take a "Goldilocks" approach to moisture within the wound bed: Not too much moisture, not too little moisture, but just the right amount of moisture balance is important to create an optimal wound healing environment.

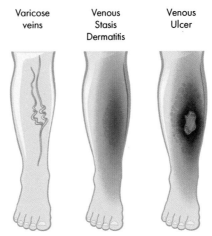

Varicose veins   Venous Stasis Dermatitis   Venous Ulcer

Venous Stasis Disease

Venous stasis is a spectrum of disease. Veins that do not move blood effectively back to the heart can become engorged causing the veins to stretch and dilate, irreversibly. You know these as varicose veins. Over time, the walls of varicose veins can become thin and 'leaky' causing fluid to actually leak out of the vein and into the tissues of the leg causing what we see as leg swelling or "edema". As edema proceeds the swelling of the legs stretches the skin and decreases blood flow to the skin leading to skin inflammation, or Venous Stasis Dermatitis. The skin inflammation of stasis dermatitis can cause small breaks in the skin which can increase your risk of skin infection (cellulitis), weeping of edema fluid from the skin, and ultimately ulceration and breakdown of the skin leading to Venous Stasis Ulcers.

Now, as we discussed earlier in this section, underlying all of these issues of fluid and drainage in venous disease is often injury to the valves of the veins. Some common mechanisms by which vein injury occurs include occupations or lifestyles that involve prolonged standing. Standing stationary for long periods of time over months and years creates a situation where the leg veins, starting from the ankle, are regularly exposed to a high-pressure state from the tall column of blood in the vein above it, trying to return to the heart. Other conditions that can create high-pressure gradients in the leg veins like this are obesity, pregnancy, trauma to the muscle or bone, and past or present blood clots within the veins.

It is also important to know that venous disease is a progressive condition, meaning that once the valves have been damaged, they cannot be fully restored to their previous normal function. This means that the best we can do is manage the symptoms and limit disease progression by controlling leg swelling and lowering pressure in the veins. I tell my patients this is best done using the following three techniques: (1) elevating the legs, (2) walking, and (3) compression therapy.

Leg elevation, using pillows or positioning cushions, is particularly effective because it helps reverse the single greatest force that exacerbates venous disease: gravity. Instead of blood having to fight gravity to slowly climb its way "uphill" back to the heart, leg elevation essentially creates a downhill slope that allows blood to simply flow back to the heart with little to no effort. While using pillows or positioners that elevate your legs above the level of the heart is ideal, elevating your feet even slightly as you sit in a chair helps reduce the pressure within the veins of the legs and the development of edema.

Similarly, walking (if you are able) helps move blood up the veins and back to the heart by recruiting muscles of the leg to act as a sort of pump. With each step, the leg muscles generate a pumping effect around the veins that helps "push" the venous blood up and along. By helping to pump the blood forward, walking works to prevent the buildup of standing pressure within the veins.

Finally, using compression therapy can be an effective way to control the symptoms and progression of venous stasis disease. Think of compression therapy as giving your legs a super-suit to fight swelling. Compression therapy is usually applied in the form of specialized compression socks (or stockings) or by using elastic compression bandages. While these therapies are not for everyone, compression therapy can help reduce swelling and pressure within the veins of the legs. In fact, I wear compression stockings every day because I'm on my feet so much for work. For me, they are great for reducing the feeling I used to have of pressure and heaviness in my legs at the end of a long workday. Different from elevation and ambulation, compression is a therapy that is applied *to* the body, so consult your medical provider prior to starting compression therapy.

That's it. Elevation. Ambulation. Compression. These three interventions are my mainstays for managing the symptoms and progression of venous stasis disease.

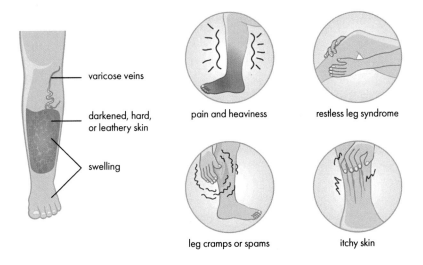

Evaluation and Treatment of Venous Disease

Treatment of venous stasis disease based on a 3-pronged approach:

1. Elevate the legs above the level of the heart whenever possible (but any elevation is better than none)

2. Ambulation - try to take short walks if and when possible. Walking uses the leg muscles to squeeze blood vessels to keep blood flowing.

3. Compression therapy - if okay with your doctor, wearing special socks or bandages that gently squeeze the legs helps the veins to work better and limit swelling.

Remember that once you have venous disease, it is a condition you will always live with, but how severely it manifests will depend on how well you can manage pressure in the veins and edema in the legs. Here are some highly effective interventions that I recommend in the management of venous stasis disease and edema:

- Leg elevation: Whenever possible, raise your legs above heart level with pillows or positioning cushions to facilitate blood flow back to the heart.

- Regular ambulation (walking): Engage in gentle walking or leg exercises to promote blood circulation and prevent blood pooling.

- Compression therapy: Use compression stockings or bandages as prescribed by your healthcare provider to improve venous return and reduce edema.

- Skincare: Keep your skin clean and moisturized, avoiding irritants and potential injuries.

- Weight management: Maintain a healthy weight to reduce the burden on your venous system.

  Avoid prolonged sitting or standing: Take breaks and change positions frequently to prevent prolonged venous stasis.

Always remember to consult with your healthcare provider for personalized guidance and recommendations to manage your venous disease. This requires a multidimensional approach, but together, you can work toward minimizing symptoms and improving your quality of life.

Surgical Wounds

Sometimes, after a surgical procedure, a wound may not heal as expected. Sometimes a wound may reopen unexpectedly, causing what we call a "non-healing surgical wound" or a "wound dehiscence." There may be a number of reasons why something like this happens. I know it sounds scary, but I see occurrences like this every day, and they are often quite treatable. Let's dive right into those reasons.

One common reason for a surgical wound separating (or dehiscing) is tension along the surgical scar. Surgical scars overlying joints or on load-bearing areas of the body could be at a higher risk of unexpectedly reopening. Examples of such surgical sites might be incisions over the knee or ankle joints or incisions on the foot or buttock. For better or worse, pain at the surgical site can actually help to limit the movement or use of these body parts to give them time to heal. Similarly, if there happens to be a lot of soft tissue swelling underneath an incision, this can also put a stretch on the skin that may increase the risk of wound separation. In certain situations, your surgeon might choose to use a splint or a cast to help reduce tension when the surgery is in or around a joint, or they may instruct you to use ice or a compression wrap to keep swelling down at the surgical site. Every surgery and surgeon is different, and this is in no way medical advice, so consult your medical provider for best practices for supporting the healing of your particular surgical wound.

Similarly, surgical sites in areas where the skin is under regular pressure, like the skin of the backside or feet, may also be at increased risk for separation from pressure and tension that pulls the healing wound edges apart. In these situations, offloading the surgical site is key to supporting wound healing. Using pillows or specialized body positioners under or around the surgical site can reduce or completely relieve unwanted pressure on the wound edges.

Sometimes, when wounds have a hard time healing, it can be due to a less than ideal blood supply to the surgical site. This is particularly true in the case of surgeries occurring in areas affected by poor circulation. Conditions like arterial disease and diabetes, as we discussed in earlier sections of this book, can wreak havoc on wound healing.

You see, when surgery is performed in an area affected by circulation problems, the tissues already have a poor blood flow environment. Then, on top of this, when a surgeon like me has to cut through tissues (including blood vessels), it further destroys some of the blood flow to the area. Existing circulation issues plus newly surgically severed blood vessels can make it even harder for oxygen and nutrients to reach a surgical wound compared to even before the surgery. For this reason, surgeons will often do extensive testing to assess the circulation of the tissue in certain high-risk individuals. Even still, complications from poor blood flow can occur, causing a wound to dehisce or fail to heal.

Infection can also play a role in delaying wound healing. Despite taking every precaution during a surgical procedure, wounds can still sometimes become seeded with bacteria, which can lead to inflammation and infection that can impair the body's ability to heal. In some cases, infections like this can cause the wound to open, resulting in a dehisced surgical wound.

Other factors, like poor nutrition and smoking, can also contribute to a non-healing or dehisced surgical wound. These, as well as other medical conditions and lifestyle choices, can cripple the body's natural healing mechanisms and make it more challenging for the wound to heal properly.

Managing non-healing surgical wounds can be complex. In some cases, additional procedures or interventions may be necessary, such as wound debridement (removal of dead or infected tissue), giving antibiotics for infection control, or using specialized wound dressings and devices. It's crucial to work closely with your healthcare provider to develop a personalized treatment plan tailored to your specific wound care needs and situation.

Wound healing can take time, so patience is also a key factor. It is important to follow your doctor's instructions regarding wound care, such as keeping the wound clean and dry, changing dressings as advised, and avoiding activities that may cause unnecessary stress to the wound bed.

Remember, the challenges in healing non-healing or dehisced surgical wounds can be multifactorial. By addressing the underlying causes, working closely with your healthcare team, and adhering to proper wound care, we can improve the chances of successful healing. If you have any concerns or notice any changes in your surgical wound, don't hesitate to reach out to your healthcare provider for guidance and support.

The Non-Healing Wound

Dealing with a wound that will not heal can be as frustrating as it is challenging. While many chronic wounds will take longer than we would like to heal, there are a small number of chronic wounds that, despite our best efforts, simply won't heal at all. Knowing this, it is so important not to lose hope. Successful long-term management of a non-healing wound can still result in a wound that is quite manageable with minimal impact on one's quality of life.

Several things can contribute to a wound's inability to heal in the face of optimized treatment. For instance, chronic conditions like diabetes and immune system disorders can impair the body's ability to heal itself. Infections, especially those that are deep-seated or antibiotic-resistant, can also slow down the healing process. Certain medications like steroids and immunosuppressive drugs can interfere with the body's natural healing processes. Furthermore, old scarring and tissue damage from an old injury, prior surgery, or radiation therapy may have damaged tissues and blood flow to a wound bed enough to prevent it from coming together and healing.

Factors That Delay Healing

The good news is that even if some wounds don't heal, there are still ways to manage and improve their condition. Regular wound monitoring and ongoing adjustments to your treatment plan based on the evolution of your wound is vital. For non-healing wounds, your healthcare provider will continue to explore alternative and advanced approaches and may involve wound care specialists, vascular surgeons, plastic surgeons, or other experts to enhance your wound management plan.

- Reduced skin and soft tissue mass (particularly with age)

- Poor nutrition or hydration

- Poor blood flow to the wound bed

- Poor function of the respiratory system (oxygen delivery)

- Poor function of the immune system

- Chronic medical conditions

- Polypharmacy (multiple medications)

- Limited mobility

- Incontinence

- Lifestyle (smoking, etc.)

- Poor adherence to medical instructions

Maintaining a positive outlook and staying proactive in your wound care regimen is crucial. Remember that every individual's healing journey is unique, and while it may take time and patience, a good healthcare team will be dedicated to supporting you throughout your healing journey. By working together and making necessary adjustments, we can achieve successful wound management and improve your quality of life.

Failure To Heal

SIGNS	CAUSES	INTERVENTIONS
Dry Wound Bed	Inadequate hydration Exposure wound to air	Hydration Use a dressing that maintains wound bed moisture
No change in size or depth over weeks OR Increase in wound size or depth	Pressure or trauma Poor nutrition / hydration Poor blood flow Poor circulation Poor control of underlying diseases (diabetes, respiratory issues) Biofim or bacteria Wound infection	Rule out local causes (ie pressure) that may limit wound healing Evaluate systemic causes and medical conditions that may limit wound healing
Necrotic Tissue	Poor Blood Flow	Consider debridement by wound care provider
Increased wound drainage or new purulent drainage	Tissues Damage Inflammation Wound Infection	Must rule out infection Absorptive wound dressings
Maceration (white skin)	Excess Moisture	Consider absorptive wound dressings and protection of skin creams
Undermining or Bruising of surrounding skin	Excess Pressure	Pad, protect, and offload area affected from pressure and shear injury

Wound Healing at the End-of-Life

Facing reality as we approach the end of someone's life can be difficult. Similarly, wound healing in the end-of-life setting can be daunting and overwhelming. Wounds occurring at this terminal stage of life may not heal, despite our best efforts and advanced medical interventions. Understanding this is crucial, but it's equally important not to lose hope. Effective and compassionate wound management can significantly improve comfort and quality of life.

Several factors can influence wound healing in end-of-life care. As we've discussed before, chronic conditions such as advanced stages of cancer, kidney failure, or heart disease can severely impair the body's natural healing processes. The body's immune response is often weakened in this stage of life, making it harder to fight infections that can delay healing. Medications commonly used in palliative care, like steroids and chemotherapy agents, can also impede wound healing. Additionally, reduced mobility and nutritional deficits can further complicate the situation, as the body struggles to repair itself.

However, there are strategies to manage these wounds effectively. Regular assessment and meticulous care can prevent further complications and alleviate discomfort. This often involves a team of healthcare professionals, including wound care specialists, palliative care doctors, and nurses, who can provide tailored care plans. Advanced wound care techniques, such as specialized dressings, negative pressure wound therapy, and pain management strategies, can play a crucial role in maintaining comfort and dignity.

Staying positive and engaged in the care process is essential. Everyone's journey is unique, and adapting care plans to meet individual needs and preferences is key. By focusing on comfort and quality of life, and through the support of a dedicated healthcare team, it is possible to manage wounds effectively, ensuring that the patient remains as comfortable as possible during this challenging transition.

IV. Treating Your Wounds

Wound Healing Basics

Whether we're dealing with a new straightforward wound or a lingering chronic one, at the end of the day, your body needs to figure out how to heal itself. We can certainly support wound healing, and we can optimize wound treatments, but it is the body's response to injury—like inflammation and granulation—that is ultimately responsible for closing and healing a wound.

As we mentioned before, the body's natural healing processes are often compromised in the case of chronic wounds. Problems like decreased mobility, diabetes, anemia, poor nutrition, and circulation issues—to name a few—can stack the deck against us as we try to heal chronic wounds. While these kinds of issues can certainly pose a challenge, they are usually not complete barriers to healing. By understanding how physical and medical issues prevent healing, we can start to look for ways to minimize the effects of these issues and, in some cases, even completely work around them. Medical advancements, special procedures, and specific treatments may help our cause, but, ultimately, we really do have to rely on the body's own ability to heal itself. There's simply no substitute for the healing power that's written in our genes. It's our job to support the body's effort to heal itself by coming up with a plan to tip the balance of healing in our favor—from the side of chronic underlying conditions back to the side of wound health and wound healing.

A Holistic Approach

First and foremost, to heal chronic wounds, we need to understand that wound management extends beyond just the wounds we see with our eyes.

Wound healing requires a holistic approach—one that involves addressing the physical, medical, and environmental issues surrounding the wound. As a wound care specialist, I believe a holistic approach that embraces the entire well-being of the patient is at the very center of fostering wound health and wound healing. Here's what you need to know.

1. Contamination and Infection

Effective infection control is a critical aspect of managing chronic wounds. Left unchecked, wound infections can be devastating to the healing process and lead to severe complications. By using stringent infection control measures, you can greatly reduce the risk of complications and accelerate the healing process.

Understanding the signs of infection, implementing proper wound cleansing techniques, and following appropriate infection prevention measures are essential for successful wound management. So, let's equip you with some principles and guidelines to ensure that you and your caregivers can effectively prevent and address infections.

Early signs of infection can include increased pain at the wound site. It may start to feel more tender or sensitive than before, and you might also notice redness around the wound that spreads or worsens over time. Another early sign, though harder to interpret, is increased drainage from a wound bed. Finally, there will be increased warmth around the wound—that is, the wound and the skin immediately around it are hotter than the surrounding skin.

Late signs of infection are more concerning and may call for immediate medical attention. One of the late signs is the presence of pus or a thick, yellowish fluid coming from the wound. Pus can have a strong smell and may be a sign that bacteria in the wound bed is causing an infection. Additionally, if you notice an increase in new swelling around the wound, this could also be a late sign of infection. Swelling may cause the area to feel tight or look puffy.

It is important to realize that a wound infection doesn't look like just one thing. It represents a clinical picture made up of varying combinations of findings, so identifying only one of the signs or symptoms above may or may not represent an actual wound infection. Still, it is vitally important that you continually take inventory of the appearance of your wound. If you experience two or more of the early signs mentioned above or just one of the late signs of infection mentioned above, it's important to contact your healthcare provider for further evaluation and recommendations. Remember, when it comes to wound complications, early detection and prompt intervention are key for preventing wound deterioration and fostering healing.

2. Offloading, Elevation, and Repositioning

While contamination and infection can be one of the biggest roadblocks to wound healing, wound offloading and body repositioning can be one of your best allies in trying to heal your wound. By "repositioning," I mean redistributing your body weight on a regular basis to continuously redistribute pressure around your wound site. By "offloading," I mean using one or more pillows or using a body positioner like a cushioned wedge, donut, or padded booties to help take pressure off your wound. Studies show that proper offloading significantly improves wound healing outcomes, so it is important to understand why.

As we discussed when talking about pressure wounds, when you have continuous pressure on an area of skin or on a wound, you can end up disrupting blood flow to that tissue, causing worsening tissue damage. Excessive pressure can have the same effect on diabetic, venous, and other wound types as well. Therefore, no matter what type of wound you have, it's important to optimize circulation to the area for a more optimal healing environment for your wound.

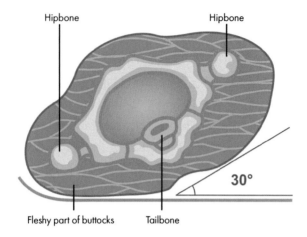

Hipbone

Hipbone

30°

Fleshy part of buttocks   Tailbone

Offloading and Repositioning

Pressure injury prevention and treatment are centered on offloading pressure points and regular patient repositioning side-to-side to alleviate sustained trauma to these areas. With repositioning the idea is to alternate resting the patient's body weight alternatingly one buttock or the other. This reduces direct pressure on the hip bones and tailbone where pressure injury is most likely. Patient repositioning is critical for minimizing tissue damage due to limited mobility.

Positioning

Often, fashioning pillows or ideally a body wedge (if you have one) can help a patient maintain a proper offloading position in bed with the hip bone approximately 30 degrees off the bed or chair they are in.

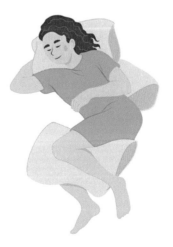

Let's talk about bed repositioning first. If you're someone confined to the bed for long periods of time, it's a good idea to change your body position every couple of hours. For instance, you can start by lying on your back for two hours, then turn onto one side for another two hours, and then finally switch to the other side for the next two hours. Repeating this schedule can help redistribute pressure more evenly across your body parts and reduce the risk of developing or worsening an ulcer.

When it comes to sitting in a chair, it's best to limit the amount of time you spend in that position. Prolonged sitting can put pressure on certain areas and increase the injury risk for new and existing pressure ulcers. As a general guideline, try to avoid sitting in the same position in the same chair for longer than one hour at a time. If possible, it's a good idea to take breaks and move around a bit before returning to a seated position.

Now, let's discuss some tools that can help with repositioning and protecting vulnerable areas:

- Chair cushions: These are specially designed cushions that provide extra support and cushioning for your buttocks and back when sitting in a chair. They help distribute pressure and reduce the risk of developing pressure ulcers.

- Heel boots: These are soft, padded boots that are worn on the feet to protect the heels from pressure and friction. They are particularly useful for individuals who spend a lot of time in bed or who have limited mobility.

- Leg elevators: These are foam or inflatable cushions that elevate your legs, helping to relieve pressure on the heels, calves, and lower back. They are especially beneficial for individuals with severe mobility limitations.

- Body wedges: These are triangular-shaped cushions that can be used to support different parts of the body, such as the back, hips, or legs.

They help maintain proper body alignment and relieve pressure on specific areas.

Among these tools, I highly recommend leg elevators and body wedges for individuals with severely limited mobility. For example, if you have a pressure wound on your lower back, I often recommend using a wedge-shaped cushion for the bed or a donut-shaped cushion for your chair to relieve the pressure on that specific area of the body when sitting or lying down. Positioners provide excellent support to help treat and protect the more vulnerable areas like the feet, heels, sacrum, and back. They can significantly aid in the healing and prevention of wounds, so I cannot recommend them enough for my patients.

In fact, I generally suggest that anyone with a chronic wound and any mobility limitations use some type of designated pillow, positioner, or offloading device. Even if you don't have a wound right now, using such devices as a preventive measure can help reduce the risk of developing pressure wounds in the future.

Remember, offloading and body repositioning are simple yet very, *very* powerful techniques to support wound healing. By addressing the issues of pressure on an affected area, we can improve blood circulation, minimize tissue damage, and help your wound heal most efficiently. If you have any concerns or questions about offloading techniques, or need help with choosing the right device for you, speak with your healthcare provider to find the best solution for your particular needs.

3. Clearing Debris

Creating an optimal wound bed environment is paramount for wound healing. Factors such as moisture balance (see the discussion on "Wound Drainage," p. 58), temperature, and oxygen supply can significantly impact wound healing. By using proper wound dressings, topical treatments, and adjunct therapies, we can create an environment that fosters tissue generation and accelerates the healing process. Your wound care provider will determine the best daily wound dressings for your wound, but let's talk about the best evidence-based strategies for creating an optimal healing environment for chronic wound management.

Proper wound bed preparation involves removing non-viable tissue and promoting the growth of new, healthy granulation tissue that we need for wound healing. Good wound care providers may regularly or intermittently perform specialized procedures to clear necrotic, unhealthy, or unwanted material within the wound bed at your scheduled wound care visit.

Wound Color

RED = Resolving / Healing
Red wound indicates normal healing is proceeding with new blood vessels and healthy grannulation tissue forming within the wound bed to fill it in.

YELLOW **= Intervention / Attention Needed**
Soft, yellow slough within the wound bed is, quite simply, dead tissue. Slough creates an ideal environment for bacterial growth which increases the risk of wound infection. Therefore, slough should be cleared by your wound care provider, if possible

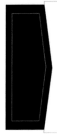
BLACK = Dead Tissue (Necrosis)
Black, necrotic tissue is the most ominous sign of poor wound healing. Necrotic tissue will not heal and will eventually be lost to auto-amputation or surgical removal. Prior to it's inevitable loss, the biggest concern with 'black' tissue is the risk of infection. Because necrotic tissue has no blood flow it can not be treated with antibiotics (which circulate in the blood). Therefore black, necrotic tissue requires a predetermined medical or surgical plan of action.

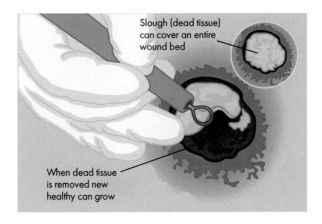

Slough (dead tissue) can cover an entire wound bed

When dead tissue is removed new healthy can grow

Necrotic Tissue and Wound Debridement

Necrotic tissue refers to 'slough' or eschar - dead tissue within the wound bed that has lost its blood supply. Necrotic tissue can impede wound healing by limiting the growth of new cells and can increase the risk of wound complications like infection.

Timely removal of necrotic tissue through sharp wound debridement is essential to facilitate optimal wound healing and minimize the risk of wound complications.

It is equally important to continue cleaning the wound between visits to your care provider. This is done with regular wound cleansings. Before applying a new bandage, it's important to clean and prepare the wound bed with every dressing change. This means gently washing and refreshing the wound bed according to your wound care provider's instructions. Depending on your particular wound, there are a variety of options for wound cleansing.

Cleaning a chronic wound is crucial for its proper healing. Follow the steps below to ensure a clean and infection-free wound care routine.

Materials Needed:

- Gloves
- Gauze sponge or pad
- Plastic trash bag

- Towel
- Saline solution or water
- Soft, clean towel

Steps to Clean:

1. Put on new gloves to maintain cleanliness and prevent the introduction of bacteria.

2. Place a towel under the body part that has the wound to catch any moisture or debris during the cleaning process.

3. Wet a gauze sponge or pad with saline solution or water. Make sure that it is damp but not dripping.

4. Starting from the center of the wound, gently clean in circular motions outward, covering an area of at least one inch beyond the wound's edge.

5. Avoid wiping from the outer edges toward the center, as this can introduce germs into the wound.

6. Clean any liquid draining from the wound.

7. Discard used gauze or cloth into a plastic trash bag.

8. Use a new gauze pad as often as necessary during the cleaning process.

9. Use a fresh gauze pad moistened with saline or water to rinse the wound and remove any loose debris not eliminated during the initial cleaning.

10. Discard all used cleaning materials, including gloves, into the plastic trash bag.

11. Pat the skin surrounding the wound gently with a soft, clean towel to ensure it is thoroughly dry.

12. Check the wound for any signs of redness, drainage, swelling, or unusual odor.

13. Observe the new tissue at the wound's bottom, which should be light red or pink and may appear lumpy or glossy. Avoid disturbing this delicate tissue, as it can bleed easily.

Wound cleansers may contain soaps, specific enzymes, and sometimes emulsifiers—all of which are designed to help break down and remove dirt, debris, and bacteria from the wound bed. The following table is a list of products your wound care doctor might choose from for cleaning and clearing your wound of debris, day-to-day.

WOUND CLEANSER	SUITABLE FOR
Normal saline solution	All types of wounds; mild to moderate severity
Hydrogen peroxide	Minor wounds; avoid in deep or chronic wounds
Iodine-based solutions	Infected wounds; not for use in deep wounds
Antibacterial ointments	Minor wounds; helps prevent infection
Hypochlorous acid solution	All types of wounds; antimicrobial properties
Wound cleansing wipes	Superficial wounds; convenient for on-the-go
Wound irrigation solutions	Deep wounds; effective for wound flushing
Silver-based dressings	Infected wounds; wounds at risk of infection
Acetic acid solution	Chronic wounds; antimicrobial properties
Collagenase ointment	Chronic wounds; aids in dead tissue removal
Wound debridement agents	Chronic wounds; helps remove dead tissue

4. Dressing the Wound

After cleaning, the next step in treating your wound is to apply one or more dressings to the wound bed. The dressings chosen by your wound care provider will depend on the type of wound you have, the wound's location, and the environmental conditions for the wound. There are all types of dressings available on the market. The following table will help you understand the different dressings your provider might prescribe for you.

TYPE OF DRESSING	SUITABLE CHRONIC WOUND TYPES
Alginate dressings	Moderate to highly draining wounds, pressure ulcers
Hydrocolloid dressings	Light to moderately draining wounds, pressure ulcers
Foam dressings	Moderate to heavily draining wounds, pressure ulcers
Hydrogel dressings	Dry or minimally draining wounds, partial-thickness burns
Transparent films	Superficial wounds, minor abrasions, surgical incisions
Collagen dressings	Chronic wounds with minimal to heavy drainage, pressure ulcers
Composite dressings	Various chronic wounds; combining multiple functions
Antimicrobial dressings	Infected chronic wounds, wounds at risk of infection
Silicone dressings	Hypertrophic scars, keloids, donor sites
Honey-impregnated dressings	Infected chronic wounds, wounds with delayed healing
Silver-impregnated dressings	Infected chronic wounds, wounds at risk of infection

Steps to Dress a Chronic Wound

To dress the wound, first start by gathering the supplies. You need to have a new dressing, tape, and clean gloves ready. Open the packaging for the new dressing, taking care to maintain its sterility by touching only the corners of the dressing. If necessary (and consistent with the manufacturer's instructions), cut the dressing to the appropriate size for the wound.

Carefully center the prepared dressing over the wound and take care that it covers the entire wound surface. Your particular wound dressing may be one of many product types: a cream, an ointment, a powder, or a sheet of some type of material. Your wound might also require using a secondary dressing to cover the first ("primary") dressing above. In any case, heed attention to your provider's wound dressing instructions and avoid aggressively disturbing the wound during your dressing changes.

Secure the wound dressing in place by using medical tape. Ensure the tape is applied firmly but not too tight, allowing for proper circulation and comfort. If using multiple pieces of tape, apply them in a crisscross pattern for added stability. Make sure that the dressing is securely in place, covering the wound adequately without any wrinkles or gaps. Confirm that the skin barrier provides a protective seal around the wound.

Carefully remove the gloves, turning them inside out as you do so avoid contamination. Dispose of the gloves in an appropriate waste container. Thoroughly wash your hands with soap and water to maintain cleanliness and reduce the risk of infection.

Daily wound cleansing is like giving your wound a spa session. It cleanses the tissues, removes debris, revitalizes tissues, and improves circulation to help prevent infection and optimize healing. Only after proper cleaning should a new dressing be applied to protect the wound and help it heal faster before putting on a fresh bandage.

5. Pain Management: Finding Comfort, Finding Relief

Pain management is a key part of the healing journey. Chronic wounds can often cause discomfort and can even limit your involvement in normal daily activities. In this section, we'll explore various pain management strategies to help alleviate pain and enhance your overall well-being.

When it comes to pain control in wound healing, our goal is not necessarily to eliminate the pain from your wound completely. Actually, pain is often a good indicator of when we are doing the right thing and when we might be doing the wrong thing. What we really want to do is to minimize the pain enough so that you can tolerate dressing changes, move around and reposition, and participate in your regular activities of daily living. To do this, we are able to use both medication-based (pharmacologic) and drug-free approaches.

For pharmacologic pain control, the aim is to use medications in a way that helps you feel more comfortable without causing excessive sedation or other negative effects. We want to strike a balance between pain relief and ensuring your overall well-being. It's important to have only one medical provider overseeing your pain management. I cannot stress this enough. This ensures a consistent treatment plan and prevents potential conflicts or complications that may arise from multiple doctors prescribing medications.

Apart from medication, there are also a variety of drug-free options for achieving pain control. These techniques can be used either alongside medication or as stand-alone strategies:

- Cold or heat therapy: Applying a cold pack or warm compress to the area can help alleviate pain and, in the case of cold therapy, may also reduce swelling.

- Elevation: Keeping the affected area raised above the level of your heart can minimize swelling and discomfort.

- Distraction techniques: Engaging in activities that divert your attention—such as listening to music, watching a movie, or reading a book—can help take your mind off the pain.

- Relaxation techniques: Practicing deep-breathing exercises, meditation, or guided imagery can promote relaxation and reduce pain perception.

- Physical therapy (PT): In some cases, performing exercises and gentle movements recommended by a physical therapist can help manage pain and improve healing. While many resources for PT are freely accessible on the internet, you should always consult a licensed physical therapist before initiating any rehabilitation plan.

- Transcutaneous electrical nerve stimulation (TENS): TENS uses pads placed on the skin to stimulate muscles and increase blood flow. It may offer an alternative way to manage pain and promote healing.

It's crucial to manage expectations regarding pain control. The goal is to minimize your discomfort and make it tolerable rather than completely eradicate it. Overmedicating (taking too much medication) can have negative effects, such as excessive drowsiness, impaired judgment, and even a dependence on the medication. That's why it is crucial to follow your prescribed medication regimen carefully and communicate any concerns regarding your pain management with your medical provider.

Remember, your providers are there to support you throughout your healing journey, and this includes management of wound-related pain. I find that patients do best when they approach pain control using both pharmacologic and non-pharmacologic methods as this strategy tends to provide them with the best pain control while also minimizing the risk of overmedication and its negative effects.

6. Nutrition and Hydration

Another very important aspect of wound management is nutrition. Proper nutrition and hydration are crucial for wound healing. When it comes to nutrition, think again of your body as a construction site—it needs the right materials to build and repair tissues. A well-balanced diet provides these building blocks, helping your body heal properly.

First and foremost, calories are incredibly important. Just getting a sufficient amount of energy (calories) in the form of food and drink is so important because those calories are the "worker bees" of the construction crew. Without energy, work at the wound bed construction site is slow and drags out over time.

Next, getting enough protein is key. Foods like lean meats, fish, eggs, beans, and dairy products are rich in protein and provide the necessary amino acids that support tissue repair and regeneration. Think of protein as the building blocks that will fill in your wound and cover it closed. Including adequate protein in your diet helps your body rebuild damaged tissues, such as skin, muscles, and blood vessels.

Also, vitamins and minerals are like the power tools that ensure everything runs as smoothly and as efficiently as possible. In particular:

- Vitamin C (found in citrus fruits and leafy greens) is essential for collagen synthesis, which is a key component in wound healing.

- Vitamin A (found in carrots, sweet potatoes, and spinach) promotes the growth of new cells.

- Zinc (present in seafood, nuts, and whole grains) plays a vital role in cell division and wound closure.

Now let's talk about hydration. Water is like the transportation system that moves all the materials where they need to go and keeps everything flowing smoothly. Staying properly hydrated supports healthy blood circulation and ensures that protein, essential nutrients, and oxygen are able to reach the wound site efficiently. Proper hydration also aids in the removal of waste products and toxins from the body, promoting overall tissue health.

To ensure that you're well hydrated, aim to drink plenty of water through-out the day. It's especially important to increase your fluid intake when you have a wound. In addition to water, you can also obtain hydration from other sources like herbal teas as well as fruits and vegetables with high water content. All that said, it is important to note here that there are a number of medical conditions that require strict control of one's water intake, so please consult with your doctor if you are considering active hydration as a part of your wound care plan.

Remember, proper nutrition and hydration provide the fuel and the tools your body needs to heal effectively. A well-balanced diet—rich in protein and essential vitamins and minerals—serves as the building blocks for tissue repair and regeneration. Adequate hydration supports healthy blood circulation and overall tissue health. By taking care of your nutrition and hydration, you're giving your body the best chance to heal optimally.

7. Mobility and Exercise: Enhancing Circulation and Healing

Physical activity and mobility play a vital role in your wound-healing journey. Engaging in appropriate exercises can do wonders for your wound healing. Let's talk about why exercise is so important and how it can help you recover.

- Exercise enhances blood circulation. When you move your body, your heart pumps blood more effectively, delivering all the necessary nutrients and oxygen to the wound site. This boost in blood flow helps your body heal faster and more efficiently.

- Exercise improves muscle strength. Strong muscles around the wound area can offer better support, protecting the healing tissue, and reducing the risk of complications. It's like having a strong support team to help your body during the healing process.

Now, how do you incorporate exercise into your routine? At first, you will want to focus on gentle range-of-motion exercises and stretching. These exercises can keep your joints flexible and prevent stiffness while being gentle on the wound. Additionally, low-impact activities such as walking and swimming can help you stay active without putting too much strain on the wound.

It's important to remember that each person's situation is unique. This is why it's essential to tailor your exercise routine to your specific wound type and overall health condition. Your healthcare provider can guide you on which exercises are best for you.

As you progress in your healing journey, it's so important to gradually increase your activity level. Listen to your body and follow your healthcare provider's recommendations. It's like taking small steps toward your goal of better healing and overall well-being.

Besides the physical benefits, exercise also contributes to your mental well-being. When you exercise, your body releases endorphins. I like to call them "feel-good" chemicals. Endorphins can boost your mood and help you stay positive during your healing process, and having a positive mindset is just like having a cheerleader encouraging you and your body to heal.

In summary, physical activity and mobility are huge allies in wound healing. They enhance blood flow, improve muscle strength, and prevent complications. By incorporating gentle range-of-motion exercises, stretching, and low-impact activities into your daily routine, you're giving your body the support it needs. Remember to tailor your exercises to your specific situation and gradually increase your activity level as you heal. Your journey to healing involves not just your body but also your mind, and exercise can contribute to your overall well-being and positive mindset.

8. Effective Communication and Shared Decision-Making

Open and honest communication is the cornerstone of any successful relationship. The same is true for the relationship between you and your healthcare provider. By fostering effective communication, you can express your concerns, preferences, and goals while your healthcare provider listens and helps you address these needs. This mutual understanding forms the foundation for shared decision-making, where you and your providers can collaborate to develop a personalized treatment plan that is tailored to your unique circumstances.

Research has shown that shared decision-making leads to increased patient satisfaction, better adherence to treatment plans, and improved health outcomes. Patients who actively participate in their care and have a voice in decision-making feel more empowered and engaged in their healing journey.

By understanding the interplay between optimizing wound bed conditions, nutrition, infection control, and a team approach, you will be equipped to provide the best possible care for your wound and your well-being.

9. Keep a Journal

Keeping a wound care journal is the easiest and best way I know of to keep track of how your wound progresses. It's a simple way to document what you notice about your wound, such as any changes in size, how it looks, and how much it hurts. This information is important because it helps you and your healthcare provider understand how well your wound is responding to treatment and can help determine if changes to the treatment plan are needed.

By writing out the wound care routine and listing daily activities in a journal, my patients often start to notice patterns in their care. They may find that a particular dressing makes the wound feel better versus a prior treatment. They may start to notice certain activities that may cause undue discomfort or may be slowing down the healing process. As a wound care doctor, these insights are extremely helpful because they allow my patients and me to have a more well-informed and insightful discussion about their care. Journaling is also another way to become a more active participant in the wound-healing process, and the more data you can provide to your wound care team, the better decisions they can make about your care.

Keeping a wound care journal will certainly give you a greater sense of control in the healing process. Plus, a journal can be a safe space to express any feelings or frustrations you might have about the process. It is very normal for chronic wound management to feel like a roller coaster ride of emotions, and a journal gives you an outlet to share those feelings. In all, keeping a wound care journal is a simple but powerful tool that can make a real difference in your wound healing experience. See the appendix of this book for a sample template of a wound care journal entry, or visit www.WoundWise.com/Journal, where you can purchase the wound care journal I have created for my own patients.

Putting Wound Healing Together

My goal in writing this book is to equip you with the knowledge and tools you need to embrace a holistic approach to wound healing. Remember, healing chronic wounds encompasses more than tending to the visible wound; it also involves addressing your overall well-being. Understanding the topics and issues we've discussed here—like nutrition, infection control, and pain management, to name a few—is where it all starts. These topics are the pieces of the jigsaw puzzle that need to come together to create an optimal healing environment.

As you put your newfound understanding into practice, you will begin to see results and gain confidence in the process that will lead you along the path to wound healing. While healing a wound can be something of a process, it is important to remember that you are not alone in this process. With the proper insights and tools, we can nearly always unlock the hidden potential for healing to bring you to a brighter, healthier future. Let's summarize what we've discussed about these chronic wounds, highlight some of the common threads among them, and develop a framework for approaching them.

It is important to understand that while we classify wounds into different categories, we must consider all your medical conditions, as a whole, when trying to heal your wounds. Other medical conditions you have can limit your wound healing or even make the wound worse. For example, if you have diabetes, the effects of a diabetic small vessel injury can compromise the blood flow needed to heal a pressure ulcer or burn. Similarly, a skin tear or surgical wound may heal more slowly if you have leg swelling from venous disease affecting the blood flow back to the heart.

To address chronic wounds effectively, therefore, we need to address the whole patient. Maximizing nutrition by following a well-balanced diet provides the building blocks necessary for tissue repair and regeneration. Engaging in physical activity and mobility—tailored to your specific wound type and overall health—enhances blood flow and tissue oxygenation, which promote healing. Quitting smoking and reducing excess weight (if these are issues) positively impact wound healing by improving blood flow and oxygen delivery, along with reducing inflammation. Finally, using specialized cushions or positioners to offload pressure from the wound area is crucial in improving tissue perfusion and minimizing damage.

It is essential for you to recognize that lifestyle interventions—nutrition, physical activity, and wound offloading—are as important to wound healing as the local dressings or interventions ordered by your wound care provider. By addressing these issues on your end, you can play an active role in optimizing your wound-healing potential.

Remember, wound healing is a complex process that requires a multi-pronged approach. By addressing compromised circulation, promoting a healthy inflammatory response, and considering all of your medical conditions, we can work together to improve your overall wound-healing outcomes.

Above all, the most important thing I want you to remember is that *you* are an active participant in your wound-healing journey and that working closely with your healthcare team will lead to the best possible outcomes for you and your chronic wound.

GLOSSARY

Abrasion – A superficial wound caused by rubbing or scraping against a rough surface.

Abscess – A localized collection of pus within tissues.

Acute Wound – A wound that heals in the expected timeframe, typically within weeks.

Adhesion – The abnormal attachment of two internal surfaces in the body.

Alginate Dressing – Absorbent dressing made from seaweed-derived fibers that absorb exudate and promote healing in heavily draining wounds.

Amino Acids – Building blocks of protein that are necessary for tissue repair.

Antimicrobial – An agent that inhibits or destroys the growth of microorganisms.

Antioxidants – Compounds that help protect cells from damage caused by free radicals, which can hinder wound healing.

Arginine – An amino acid that enhances collagen production, supports immune function, and promotes tissue repair.

Arterial Ulcer – A wound related to poor blood circulation in the arteries, typically in the legs or feet.

Atrophic – Wounds with thin or fragile tissue, often seen in elderly patients.

Autolysis – The body's natural ability to remove necrotic tissue using its own enzymes to break down devitalized tissue.

Autolytic Debridement – The body's natural process of breaking down and removing dead tissue.

Balanced Diet – A diet that includes a variety of foods from different food groups to provide all necessary nutrients.

Ballon Gastrostomy Tube (G-Tube) – A medical device inserted through the abdominal wall into the stomach and held in place by an inflatable balloon within the stomach, allowing for feeding or medication delivery in individuals who cannot eat or drink orally.

Bedridden – Being confined to a bed due to illness, injury, or physical limitations, often requiring care.

Bedsore – Also known as a pressure ulcer, is a skin injury that occurs due to prolonged pressure on the skin.

Biofilm – A protective layer formed by a community of bacteria in the wound, which can hinder healing.

Biohazard – Materials or substances that pose a risk to human health due to their biological nature, often associated with contaminated wound dressings.

Biopsy – A small piece of tissue that is removed from any part of the body for diagnostic purposes.

Blister – A raised, fluid-filled pocket that forms on the skin, typically in response to friction, heat, or irritation.

Bruise – Bleeding from broken blood vessels beneath the skin causing skin discoloration.

Callus – A hard, thickened, toughened area of skin that forms in response to repeated friction or pressure, often on the hands or feet.

Calories – Units of energy derived from food that the body needs for various functions, including wound healing.

Cancer Lesion – An abnormal growth of cells or tissue that may be cancerous, potentially posing a threat to overall health.

Carbohydrates – Macronutrients that provide energy for the body and aid in the healing process.

Chemical Debridement – Using topical agents or enzymes to break down and remove dead or necrotic tissue to promote wound healing.

Chronic Wound – A wound that does not heal in an expected timeframe, often due to underlying health issues or complications.

Clean – Wounds free from contamination or infection.

Collagen – A protein that provides strength and structure to tissue, important for wound healing.

Colonization – The presence of bacteria on the wound's surface without causing infection or harmful effects.

Compression – The use of bandages or garments to apply pressure to reduce swelling and aid circulation.

Contaminated – Wounds exposed to foreign materials or contaminants.

Contracture – Restricted range of motion of a joint, often limiting mobility.

Contusion – Commonly known as a bruise.

Debridement – The removal of dead (non-viable), foreign material or contaminated tissue from a wound to promote healing.

Deep – Wounds that extend into deeper layers of tissue.

Dehiscence – The partial or complete separation of the edges of a surgical wound.

Dermis – The thick layer of skin beneath the epidermis, containing blood vessels, nerves, and hair follicles.

Desiccation – Drying out of the wound, which can hinder healing.

Diabetic Foot Ulcer – A chronic wound commonly seen in individuals with diabetes.

Dietary Supplements – Additional nutrients or vitamins taken in the form of pills, capsules, or liquids to support nutrition.

Dietitian – A healthcare professional who specializes in nutrition and can provide guidance on dietary choices for wound healing.

Donut – A circular cushion or pad with a hole in the center, designed to surround and protect a wound.

Dressing – Material placed on a wound to protect it, absorb exudate, and promote healing.

Dressing Change – The process of removing and replacing wound dressings to assess and manage the wound.

Edema – Swelling caused by an accumulation of fluid in the tissues.

Edema Management – Techniques to reduce swelling or fluid buildup in the tissues around the wound.

Edematous – Wounds surrounded by swollen or fluid-filled tissue.

Elevation – Raising the wounded area above heart level to reduce swelling.

Enteral Nutrition – The delivery of nutrients directly into the digestive tract through methods such as tube feeding.

Epibole – When wound edges roll or fold over themselves, impeding wound healing.

Epidermis – (1) The outermost layer of skin. (2) The outer layer of the skin situated above the dermis and forms the protective barrier to the body from invading organisms.

Epithelialization – The formation of new skin cells at the wound edges to cover the wound.

Epithelializing – New skin cells forming at the edge of the wound to cover the surface in the healing process.

Epithelial Tissue – The cellular lining of the surface of the body.

Erythema – Redness of the skin often associated with inflammation.

Eschar – A thick, dry, hard, black or brown necrotic tissue that forms a scab on a wound.

Exudate – Fluid that oozes out of a wound, containing proteins, cells, and debris. Exudate can be clear, yellow, green, or bloody.

Exudative – Wounds that produce excessive drainage or exudate.

Fibrin – A protein involved in the blood clotting process.

Fistula – An abnormal connection or passageway between two organs or vessels, sometimes associated with wound complications.

Foam Dressing – A dressing with a foam-like texture that absorbs exudate, maintains a moist environment, and cushions the wound.

G-Tube – A medical device inserted through the abdominal wall into the stomach and held in place by an inflatable balloon within the stomach, allowing for feeding or medication delivery in individuals who cannot eat or drink orally.

Gangrene – Dead or dying tissue resulting from a lack of blood flow or infection.

Granulation Tissue – (1) New connective tissue formed during wound healing, characterized by a pink or beefy red appearance. (2) Facilitates wound closure in the healing process of secondary intention.

Heel Float – A technique that keeps a patient's heel elevated and suspended, preventing it from coming into contact with a surface to alleviate pressure.

Heel Protector – A specialized cushioning or support device designed to protect and offload pressure from the heels.

Hematoma – A collection of blood under the skin due to broken blood vessels often seen as a bruise or lump.

Hemostasis – (1) The process of stopping bleeding. (2) The 1st stage of wound healing where the body works to stop bleeding by constricting blood vessels and forming clots.

Hydration – Maintaining adequate fluid intake, which is crucial for wound healing.

Hydrocolloid Dressing – A type of dressing that forms a gel-like substance when in contact with wound exudate, promoting a moist wound environment.

Hyperbaric Oxygen Therapy (HBOT) – A treatment that involves breathing pure oxygen in a pressurized chamber to promote wound healing.

Hypergranulation – Excessive growth of granulation tissue above the wound surface.

Hypoxic – Wounds with reduced oxygen supply, often due to poor circulation.

Immune System – The body's defense mechanism against infections and other health threats, influenced by nutrition.

Incision – A surgical cut or wound made intentionally, typically for medical procedures.

Incontinence – Medical condition involving the loss of control over bladder and/or bowel function.

Infected – Wounds with signs of bacterial or microbial contamination.

Infection – The invasion and multiplication of microorganisms in tissues, leading to tissue damage.

Inflammation – (1) The body's natural response to injury, including wounds. (2)The 2nd stage of wound healing characterized by redness, swelling, and the activation of immune cells to defend against infection.

Iron – A vital mineral necessary for transporting oxygen in the blood which are essential for tissue oxygenation and repair.

Ischemia – Insufficient blood supply to a tissue or organ causing tissue damage and possibly wounds.

Keloid – An abnormal overgrowth of scar tissue that extends beyond the boundaries of the original wound, and tends to remain elevated and discolored.

Laceration – A wound caused by a sharp object cutting or tearing the skin.

Lean Protein Sources – Foods such as chicken, fish, beans, and tofu that provide essential protein for healing without excess fat.

Lymphedema – A swelling in the arms or legs due to a blockage or damage to the lymphatic system.

Maceration – Softening and breakdown of skin or wound tissue due to prolonged exposure to moisture.

Macrophage – A type of white blood cell that plays a key role in the inflammatory phase of wound healing.

Maggot Therapy – Applying sterile fly larvae (maggots) to a wound bed to remove dead tissue and stimulate healing.

Malabsorption – A condition where the body cannot absorb ingested nutrients properly, affecting wound healing.

Malnutrition – A condition characterized by a lack of essential nutrients in the diet, which can impair wound healing.

Malodorous – Wounds with a foul or unpleasant odor.

MASD – Moisture-Associated Skin Damage. Refers to skin injuries caused by prolonged exposure to moisture, such as from urine or sweat.

Maturation – The 4th stage of wound healing focuses on strengthening and remodeling the healed tissue to regain its strength and flexibility over time.

Minerals – Essential micronutrients (e.g., zinc, iron) that play a role in wound healing and tissue repair.

Necrosis – Death of cells or tissues, often seen as black or dark-colored areas in the wound.

Necrotic – (1) Wounds with dead or decaying tissue. (2) Dead tissue.

Negative Pressure Wound Therapy (NPWT) – A wound management technique that uses suction to promote healing.

Non-Adherent Dressing – A type of dressing that does not stick to the wound, reducing trauma during dressing changes.

Non-compliant – Wounds that result from patient non-adherence to treatment plans.

Nutrition – The process of providing the body with the necessary nutrients through food to support overall health and wound healing.

Offloader – A device or aid designed to relieve pressure and promote healing.

Offloading – Reducing pressure on affected areas to facilitate healing, often using a specialized device or technique.

Osteomyelitis – (1) Infection of the bone. (2) A severe bone infection characterized by inflammation and damage to bone tissue often caused by bacteria.

Painful – Wounds causing discomfort or pain to the patient.

Parenteral Nutrition – The intravenous delivery of nutrients when the digestive system cannot be used.

PEG Tube (Percutaneous Endoscopic Gastrostomy Tube) – A medical device inserted through the abdominal wall into the stomach via endoscopy, allowing for feeding or medication delivery in individuals who cannot eat or drink orally.

Periwound – (1) The area of skin surrounding a wound. (2) The outer margin of a wound.

Positioner – A specialized device or tool used to properly align and support a patient's body or limbs.

Pressure Reducing – Equipment used to reduce pressure on an area by supporting as much of the body surface as possible.

Pressure Ulcer – A localized injury to the skin and underlying tissue caused by prolonged pressure, shear, or friction. Often seen in bedridden or otherwise mobility-limited patients.

Primary Intention – The surgical closure of a wound with sutures or staples to promote rapid and organized healing with minimal scarring.

Proliferation – The 3rd stage of wound healing involves the formation of new tissue and blood vessels to repair the wound.

Prone – Lying face-down.

Protein – A macronutrient essential for tissue repair and the formation of new skin cells.

Puncture Wound – A wound caused by a sharp object piercing the skin.

Repositioning – The practice of regularly changing a patient's body or limb position to relieve pressure on specific areas.

RICE – Stands for Rest, Ice, Compression, and Elevation. A method used to reduce swelling and discomfort in the early stages of wound management.

Scab – A thin, crusty protective layer that forms over a wound composed of dried blood, tissue, and immune system cells.

Scalpel - A surgical instrument used for precise cutting or incisions.

Scar Tissue - Fibrous tissue that forms as a wound heals, often leaving a mark.

Secondary Intention - A natural healing process where a wound is left open to granulate and heal from the bottom up, often used for deeper or infected wounds.

Seroma - A collection of serous fluid that accumulates in a surgical wound.

Sharp Debridement - When dead or infected tissue is removed using sharp instruments such as scalpels or scissors to promote healing.

Silver Dressing - A dressing infused with silver to help prevent or manage wound infections.

Sinus Tract - A narrow, abnormal passageway leading from an abscess or cavity to the skin surface.

Skin Graft - Surgical transplantation of healthy skin to cover a wound.

Skin Substitute - Artificial or bioengineered materials used to promote tissue growth and wound closure.

Skin Tear - A traumatic injury to the skin characterized by the separation of the top layer of skin from the underlying tissue.

Slough - Soft, yellowish or whitish necrotic (dead) tissue that may be present in a wound bed.

Stasis Ulcer - A chronic wound that occurs due to poor venous circulation.

Sterile – Free from bacteria and other microorganisms.

Stitching – The process of closing a wound with sutures (stitches).

Subcutaneous Tissue – The layer of fat and connective tissue beneath the skin consisting of fat, blood vessels, and nerves providing insulation and cushioning for the body.

Superficial – Wounds affecting only the top layers of skin.

Supine – Lying face-up.

Supplemental Nutrition – The use of nutritional supplements (e.g., protein shakes) to meet dietary needs during healing.

Surgical Site Infection – An infection that develops at the site of a surgical wound.

Sutures – Stitches or other materials used to hold wound edges together during healing.

Tissue Necrosis – Death of tissue cells due to injury or disease.

Tissue Viability – The ability of tissue to survive and thrive, important in wound healing.

Topical Antibiotics – Antibiotics applied directly to the wound to prevent or treat infection.

Transparent Film Dressing – A clear, adhesive dressing that allows visualization of the wound while protecting it from outside contaminants.

Trauma – Wounds caused by injury.

Tunneling – Narrow channels extending from the wound bed into surrounding tissue.

Ulcer – A sore on the skin or mucous membrane, often due to poor circulation or pressure.

Undermining – The formation of a pocket or ledge beneath the intact skin at the wound edge.

Vascular Insufficiency – Poor blood flow to a particular area, affecting wound healing.

Venous Hypertension – A condition of elevated pressure in the veins, often in the legs, causing symptoms such as swelling and skin changes.

Venous Stasis Ulcer – (1) A chronic wound often associated with swelling (or edema). (2) A chronic wound that typically occurs in the lower leg due to poor blood circulation in the veins.

Vitamins – Essential micronutrients that support various bodily functions, including wound healing (e.g., vitamin C, vitamin D).

Wedge – A cushion or support shaped like a small incline used to offload pressure and elevate a specific area of the body.

Weight Management – Maintaining a healthy body weight, which can impact wound healing.

Wound Assessment – The evaluation of a wound's size, depth, appearance, and healing progress.

Wound Assessment Tools - Instruments and methods used by healthcare providers to measure and document wound characteristics.

Wound Bed Preparation - The process of optimizing the wound environment to promote healing.

Wound Bed - The base or bottom of the wound where new tissue forms.

Wound Dehiscence - The separation or bursting open of a previously closed wound.

Wound Documentation - Keeping records of wound assessment, treatment, and progress.

Wound Edge - The outer border of the wound.

Wound Exudate - The fluid that escapes from a wound; it may be serous, sanguineous, or purulent.

Wound Healing Stages - The process of wound healing, typically divided into 4 stages - hemostasis, inflammation, proliferation, and then maturation.

Wound Infection - The invasion and multiplication of harmful microorganisms (bacteria, fungi) in a wound, causing an inflammatory response.

Wound Irrigation - The process of rinsing a wound with a sterile solution to clean and remove debris.

Wound VAC (Vacuum-Assisted Closure) - A device that uses negative pressure (suction) to promote wound healing by removing excess fluid and promoting tissue growth.

Zinc - A mineral that promotes cell growth, collagen formation, and immune function in wound healing as well as a component of many body systems.

This glossary provides a comprehensive list of terms commonly used in wound care. Use this glossary as a reference to help you navigate conversions and counseling regarding your wound care and treatments.

APPENDIX 1
Stages of Pressure Injury

Stage 1: Non-blanchable (sustained) skin redness over a pressure point.

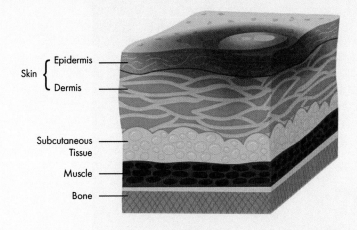

Skin { Epidermis
Dermis

Subcutaneous Tissue

Muscle

Bone

Stage 2: Damage to but not through the skin over a pressure point.

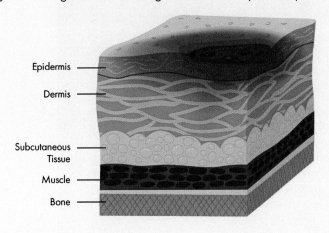

Epidermis

Dermis

Subcutaneous Tissue

Muscle

Bone

Stage 3: Damage through the skin exposing fat or subcutaneous tissue.

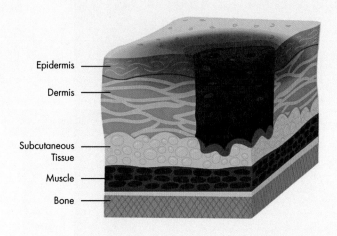

Epidermis

Dermis

Subcutaneous
Tissue

Muscle

Bone

Stage 4: Damage that exposes muscle, tendon and/or bone.

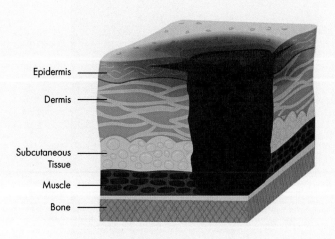

Epidermis

Dermis

Subcutaneous
Tissue

Muscle

Bone

Deep Tissue Pressure Injury: Damage to deep tissue, but overlying skin remains intact.

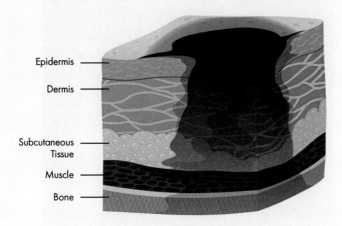

Epidermis

Dermis

Subcutaneous
Tissue

Muscle

Bone

Unstageable Pressure Injury: Open wound with necrotic (nonviable) tissue covering the healable (viable) tissue.

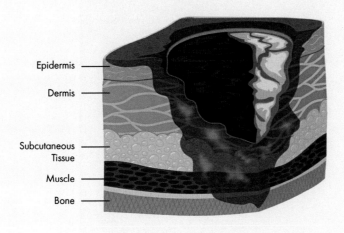

Epidermis

Dermis

Subcutaneous
Tissue

Muscle

Bone

APPENDIX 2
Wound Care Dressings

Clinical Indications:

The following dressings are commonly used in wound care for various clinical indications. Please consult your wound care provider for specific guidance on dressing selection and administration.

1 Non-Adherent Dressings:

- Telfa® Non-Adherent Dressing

- Adaptic® Non-Adhering Dressing

- Mepitel® Non-Adherent Silicone Dressing

Indicated for wounds with delicate or fragile tissue, minimizing trauma during dressing changes.

2 Transparent Films:

- Tegaderm™ Transparent Film Dressing

- Opsite™ Transparent Adhesive Film Dressing

- Bioclusive™ Transparent Film Dressing

Suitable for superficial wounds, providing a moist healing environment while allowing visualization of the wound.

3 Hydrocolloid Dressings:

- DuoDERM® Extra Thin Dressing

- Comfeel® Plus Transparent Hydrocolloid Dressing

- Tegasorb® Thin Hydrocolloid Dressing

Ideal for shallow to moderately deep wounds, promoting autolytic debridement and providing a moist healing environment.

4 Foam Dressings:

- Allevyn™ Foam Dressing

- Mepilex® Border Foam Dressing

- PolyMem® Foam Dressing

Effective for moderate to highly exudating wounds, providing absorption and cushioning while maintaining a moist wound bed.

5 Alginate Dressings:

- Algisite® M Calcium Alginate Dressing

- Kaltostat® Calcium Sodium Alginate Dressing

- Maxorb® Extra Alginate Wound Dressing

Indicated for highly exudating wounds, absorbing and retaining fluid while conforming to the wound surface.

6 Hydrogel Dressings:

- Curasol™ Hydrogel Wound Dressing

- Solosite® Gel Wound Dressing

- Intrasite® Gel Amorphous Hydrogel

Suitable for dry to minimally exudating wounds, providing moisture and promoting autolytic debridement.

7 Antimicrobial Dressings:

- Acticoat™ Antimicrobial Barrier Dressing

- Silvercel® Antimicrobial Alginate Dressing

- Mepilex® Ag Antimicrobial Foam Dressing

- Hydorfera Blue® Antimicrobial Foam Dressing

Indicated for infected wounds or wounds at risk of infection, incorporating antimicrobial agents to help control bacterial growth.

8 Compression Dressings:

- Profore® Multi-Layer Compression Bandage System

- Coban™ 2 Layer Compression System

- SurePress™ High Compression Bandage

Used for venous leg ulcers or edema management, applying controlled pressure to aid in venous return.

9 Negative Pressure Wound Therapy (NPWT):

- V.A.C.® Therapy System

- PICO™ Single-Use Negative Pressure Wound Therapy System

- Renasys™ GO Negative Pressure Wound Therapy System

Utilized for complex wounds, applying negative pressure to promote wound healing and remove excess fluid.

Please Note:

This is a representative sample list of wound care dressings and does not imply endorsement or representation of any specific dressing over another. Dressing selection should be based on individual patient needs and wound characteristics. Always consult your wound care provider for guidance regarding the selection and administration of wound dressings specific to your condition.

APPENDIX 3
Wound Care Product List

The following is a representative sample list of commonly used wound care products. Please consult your wound care provider for specific recommendations and guidance on product selection and usage.

1 Wound Cleansers:

- Saline Solution: Sterile saltwater used to gently cleanse wounds without damaging healthy tissue.

- Antiseptic Solution: Topical solutions containing antiseptic agents such as povidone-iodine (Betadine), Dakin's Solution, or chlorhexidine used to clean wounds and reduce the risk of infection.

- Non-Cytotoxic Wound Cleansers: Specialized cleansers designed to remove debris and maintain a moist wound environment without causing harm to healthy cells.

2 Topical Antibiotics:

- Bacitracin Ointment: An over-the-counter antibiotic ointment used to prevent infection in minor cuts, scrapes, and burns.

- Neomycin Ointment: An antibiotic ointment used for the prevention and treatment of superficial skin infections.

- Silver-based Ointments: Ointments containing silver ions or compounds with antimicrobial properties, used for infected wounds or wounds at risk of infection.

3 Moisturizers and Barrier Creams:

- Emollient Creams: Hydrating creams that help soften and moisturize dry, damaged skin surrounding the wound.

- Skin Barrier Creams: Products that provide a protective barrier over the skin, guarding against moisture, irritants, and friction.

4 Negative Pressure Wound Therapy (NPWT) Devices:

- V.A.C.® Therapy System: A device that applies negative pressure to the wound, promoting healing and reducing excess fluid.

- PICO™ Single-Use NPWT System: A compact, portable system that provides negative pressure wound therapy for smaller wounds.

5 Compression Bandages:

- Elastic Compression Bandages: Stretchable bandages used to apply compression for venous leg ulcers or edema management.

- Unna Boot: A semi-rigid compression dressing, often impregnated with zinc oxide and calamine, used for the management of venous stasis ulcers.

6 Skin Substitutes:

These are specialized products for specific wound types that aim to promote wound healing by providing a cellular scaffold or growth factors

- Synthetic Skin Grafts: Artificial materials that provide a temporary covering for partial-thickness wounds, promoting wound healing.

- Xenografts: Grafts derived from animal sources, used as temporary wound coverings to protect the wound bed.

Please Note:

This list is not exhaustive and serves as a general reference guide. Individual wound characteristics and patient needs may require specific product recommendations. Always consult your wound care provider for personalized advice regarding wound care product selection and usage.

APPENDIX 4
Other Wound Care Resources

Heal Your Wound is a comprehensive overview of what patients should know about chronic wound management. However, in many ways it only scratches the surface of all there is to know in wound care. The following is a list of resources related to wound care I use myself including organizations, websites, apps, books, and social media platforms. This is not an exhaustive list and the inclusion here does not imply any affiliation or endorsement. Always independently verify the credibility of sources before using them, and always seek professional medical advice from a qualified healthcare provider for personalized wound care recommendations.

Organizations:

1. **Wound, Ostomy, and Continence Nurses Society (WOCN Society)** – A professional nursing society dedicated to wound, ostomy, and continence care, providing education, resources, and support for healthcare professionals and patients. Website: www.wocn.org

2. **American Academy of Wound Management (AAWM)** – A multidisciplinary organization focused on promoting the science and practice of wound care. Website: www.aawm.org

3. **National Pressure Injury Advisory Panel (NPIAP)** – An organization dedicated to the prevention and management of pressure injuries, providing evidence-based guidelines and educational materials. Website: www.npiap.com

Websites:

1. **WoundSource** - An online wound care resource offering articles, product information, and educational materials for healthcare professionals and patients. Website: www.woundsource.com

2. **MedlinePlus** - A service of the U.S. National Library of Medicine, providing reliable information on wound care, health conditions, and treatments. Website: medlineplus.gov

3. **Mayo Clinic** - A reputable healthcare website offering wound care information, treatment options, and self-care tips. Website: www.mayoclinic.org

Apps:

1. **WoundCareAdvisor** - A mobile app designed for healthcare professionals, providing wound care guidelines, assessment tools, and educational content.

2. **WoundRounds®** - A mobile app for healthcare facilities, assisting in wound assessment, documentation, and tracking of wound healing progress.

3. **Healiant Wound** - An app for patients and caregivers, offering wound care education, tips, and reminders for wound dressing changes.

Books:

1. **Wound Care Essentials: Practice Principles (4th Edition) by Sharon Baranoski, Elizabeth A. Ayello** - A comprehensive guide covering wound assessment, treatment, and evidence-based practice.

② **Chronic Wound Care: A Problem-Based Learning Approach by Diane Krasner** - A practical book focusing on chronic wound management, including case studies and treatment strategies.

③ **Wound Care Made Incredibly Visual! (3rd Edition) by Lippincott Williams & Wilkins** - A visually engaging guide with illustrations and diagrams, making wound care concepts easy to understand.

Social Media Platforms:

① **Wound Care Education Institute (WCEI)** - Provides wound care education and resources on platforms such as Facebook, Twitter, and LinkedIn.

② **WoundSource** - Shares wound care articles, tips, and educational content on social media platforms like Facebook and Twitter.

Educational Resources:

① **Wound Care Certification Courses** - Offered by various organizations, such as WOCN Society and WoundSource, providing comprehensive wound care education and certification programs.

② **Webinars and Online Courses** - Numerous online platforms and organizations offer webinars and courses on various wound care topics, providing in-depth education and training.

APPENDIX 5
Personal Wound Care Journal

Journal entries like the one below are designed for personal use and to help facilitate communication with our doctor. Feel free to share information from your wound care journal with your care provider during appointments to help with collaborative wound management and decision-making. Avoid measuring and recording objective data, as determinations or wound progress should always be performed by your wound care provider.

Personal Wound Care Journal Template:

[Date: _____]

Observations:

(Note any changes, appearance, or sensations related to the wound. This can include size, color, pain level, drainage, and any other noticeable characteristics.)

_____

_____

Wound Care Routine:

(Describe the wound care steps performed during the day, such as cleansing, applying dressings, using topical treatments, and any other interventions.)

_____

_____

HEAL YOUR WOUND

Daily Activities:

(List any physical activities or events that may have affected the wound or the healing process.)

_____

_____

Notes and Feelings:

(Express any feelings or thoughts related to the wound care journey, including challenges, progress, or achievements.)

_____

_____

Questions for Healthcare Provider:

(Jot down any questions or concerns you would like to discuss with your wound care provider during the next appointment.)

_____

_____

Next Appointment (Date/Time): _____

Find my full format, 12-month guided wound care journal at www.WoundWise.com/journal. The Wound Care Journal is perfectly designed to help you track your wound, better engage with your provider, and manage your healthcare appointments.

NOTES

NOTES

NOTES

REFERENCES

- Wound Management Institute:
  https://www.woundheal.org/

- Wound Healing - StatPearls - NCBI Bookshelf:
  https://www.ncbi.nlm.nih.gov/books/NBK535406/

- Chronic Wounds - American Academy of Family Physicians:
  https://www.aafp.org/pubs/afp/issues/2020/0201/p159.html
  https://www.ncbi.nlm.nih.gov/books/NBK499887/

- The Global Wound Care Market to 2027:
  https://www.thebusinessresearchcompany.com/Illustrations
  https://www.ncbi.nlm.nih.gov/books/NBK441980/
  https://www.ncbi.nlm.nih.gov/books/NBK535406/
  https://www.kenhub.com/en/library/anatomy/histology-of-the-skin
  https://diabetes.org/

- Management of diabetic foot ulcers:
  https://diabetesjournals.org/compendia/article-abstract/doi/10.2337/db2020-01/144938

- The Role of Hyperglycemia in Delayed Wound Healing: A Review of the Literature:
  https://www.ncbi.nlm.nih.gov/pmc/articles/PMC7243111/
  https://www.ncbi.nlm.nih.gov/books/NBK537328/

- National Pressure Injury Advisory Panel (NPIAP):

  https://npiap.com/

  https://www.ncbi.nlm.nih.gov/books/NBK557868/

  https://www.upmc.com/services/wound-healing/conditions-we-treat/
  pressure-ulcers

- Wounds International:

  https://woundsinternational.com/

- American Professional Wound Care Association (APWCA):

  https://www.apwca.org/

INDEX

About the Author

Dr. Alvin May is a general surgeon and wound care physician serving the Southern California area for over ten years. He is a graduate of Harvard Medical School and trained in general surgery at the Boston Medical Center. Shortly after starting his career, Dr. May helped launch a national wound care company providing physician-directed wound care services to nursing homes and long-term care facilities.

In 2022, Dr. May founded MEND Wound Care, providing high-quality wound care to patients throughout the greater Los Angeles area. Compelled to reach even more patients with a message of healing, he began creating a series of educational resources and tools for patients and caregivers dealing with the day-to-day challenges of chronic wound management.

Made in the USA
Las Vegas, NV
09 May 2025

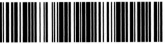

21914178R00086